A PLUME BOOK

ALL YOU NEED TO BE IMPOSSIBLY FRENCH

HELENA FRITH POWELL is a regular contributor to the *Sunday Times* (London), as well as the *Daily Mail* (London), the *Sunday Telegraph* (London), the *Tatler*, *Harpers & Queen*, and *The Independent on Sunday* (London). She lives with her husband and their five children in the Languedoc region of the south of France.

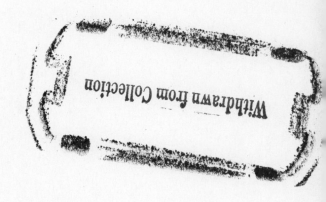

ALSO BY HELENA FRITH POWELL

More France Please

All You Need to Be Impossibly French

A Witty Investigation into the Lives, Lusts, and Little Secrets of French Women

HELENA FRITH POWELL

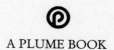

A PLUME BOOK

PLUME
Published by Penguin Group
Penguin Group (USA) Inc., 375 Hudson Street, New York, New York 10014, U.S.A.
Penguin Group (Canada), 90 Eglinton Avenue East, Suite 700, Toronto, Ontario, Canada
M4P 2Y3 (a division of Pearson Penguin Canada Inc.)
Penguin Books Ltd., 80 Strand, London WC2R 0RL, England
Penguin Ireland, 25 St. Stephen's Green, Dublin 2, Ireland (a division of Penguin Books Ltd.)
Penguin Group (Australia), 250 Camberwell Road, Camberwell, Victoria 3124, Australia
(a division of Pearson Australia Group Pty. Ltd.)
Penguin Books India Pvt. Ltd., 11 Community Centre, Panchsheel Park,
New Delhi – 110 017, India
Penguin Books (NZ), 67 Apollo Drive, Rosedale, North Shore 0632,
New Zealand (a division of Pearson New Zealand Ltd.)
Penguin Books (South Africa) (Pty.) Ltd., 24 Sturdee Avenue, Rosebank, Johannesburg
2196, South Africa

Penguin Books Ltd., Registered Offices: 80 Strand, London WC2R 0RL, England

Published by Plume, a member of Penguin Group (USA) Inc. Originally published in Great
Britain by Gibson Square Publishers.

First American Printing, December 2006
20   19   18   17   16   15   14   13

Copyright © Helena Frith Powell, 2006
All rights reserved

Ⓟ REGISTERED TRADEMARK—MARCA REGISTRADA

LIBRARY OF CONGRESS CATALOGING-IN-PUBLICATION DATA
Powell, Helena Frith.
    All you need to be impossibly French : a witty investigation into the lives, lusts, and little
secrets of French women/Helna Frith Powell.
        p. cm.
    Includes index.
    ISBN 978-0-452-28778-5
    1. Women—France—Social life and customs. 2. Lifestyles—France. 3. Beauty, Personal—
France. I. Title.

HQ1613.P69 2006
305.40944—dc22   2006040615

Printed in the United States of America

For Olivia and Bea,

French women of the future.

Contents

Two Lipsticks …   1

1. The Myth of French Style   5
2. Zen Exercise   23
3. The Secret Weapon   37
4. Never Mind the Botox   53
5. Indispensable Allies   65
6. *La Reine du Beige*   85
7. Beyond One's Control   105
8. *Bonjour paresse*   121
9. *Le Bébé surprise*   137
10. Ten Kilos   157
11. Text Appeal   173
12. Dangerous Liaisons   199

My Year in Training   217

All You Need to Be
Impossibly French

Two Lipsticks ...

The first time I visited Paris I stayed with a dancer come stripper who worked at the Lido Nightclub. I was twelve years old. My father, in those days still a handsome charmer, had arranged to meet me there for the Easter holidays. He lived in Italy but was travelling to meet me via the South of France. When I arrived at his hotel in Paris, I was told he was not there, but that the concierge had a telegram for me. It was from him: 'Have been delayed by a bottom in St Tropez. Call Sophie. Stay with her until I get there.' I asked the concierge to call the number on the telegram and spoke to Sophie. She told me that my father had arranged everything with her and to get a taxi to an address which she gave to the concierge.

I was furious when I got into the cab. What was he

thinking sending me off to some woman I had never met? Who was she anyway? Undoubtedly another one of his many girlfriends. My parents had been divorced for years, but his libertine behaviour maddened me nonetheless. When I got there, Sophie was waiting outside her apartment on the rue du Bac. She must have been in her early twenties, but to me she looked incredibly grown up and glamorous. She was tall and thin, her dark hair cut in a classic Parisian-style bobbed haircut. She wore red lipstick, jeans and a black polo-neck top. When I got out of the car, she threw her arms around me and kissed me. Being an English-educated girl, this surprised me, but I followed her into her apartment anyway.

Sophie lived in a one-bedroom studio which was incredibly Zen. She had some plants and a picture of Audrey Hepburn on the wall. There was a tiny balcony which looked out over the rue du Bac below. I didn't know who Audrey Hepburn was, but thought they looked very similar. In fact Sophie looked to me totally perfect. Slim, incredibly pretty, elegant and sophisticated. Exactly how I'd imagined a French woman should be. As the young heroine Cécile says of Anne Larsen in Françoise Sagan's novel *Bonjour Tristesse*: 'To her I owed my first glimpse of elegance.'

I stayed with Sophie for three days while waiting for my father. She worked at night, so didn't get up until midday. We spent the afternoons together, leading an almost

Claudine-style existence. Me as Colette's heroine Claudine and Sophie as Mademoiselle Aimée, the teacher she develops a crush on. I loved her clothes and look: she was always perfectly turned out. She seemed to me like a film star. I idolised her in the way a little girl idolises a fairy princess. Even when she first woke up, Sophie would look impossibly elegant in her cashmere dressing gown and hair loosely tied up. I was also astounded by the amount of time she spent covering her body and face with lotions. I had never seen a bathroom with so many magical-looking bottles. I must have driven her mad asking what every single one was.

'You don't really need all this,' she told me one day. 'All you really need to be a French woman are two lipsticks and a lover.' I asked her why two lipsticks and she looked at me in amazement. 'One for the day and the other for the evening of course.' I was too embarrassed to ask about the lover.

A few months after I went home, the image of Sophie with all her elegance faded. It wasn't until I moved to France a few years ago that I started to think about her again and realise that if I was ever going to fit in I was going to have to become more like Sophie. Although our move had gone well and we were very happy, we were always referred to as 'The English on the hill.' I realised that it wasn't just our accents that set us apart. I looked different from the women around me. I simply wasn't as stylish. Whatever it was they had, I hadn't got it.

When we still lived in England, I thought I looked pretty good. In no way did I think my style was vulgar or tacky, that my skirts were too short, my legs too hairy or my shoes too cheap. But after a few months in France I realised that I stood out as a foreigner in every way. I had to change if I was ever going to be accepted in my new country.

But where to start?

1
The Myth of French Style

'Style is life! It is the very life-blood of thought!'
Gustave Flaubert

It is the end of term at the local village primary school. The sun is shining and there is a light breeze. The parents, teachers and pupils are gathered under the plane trees in the playground. My daughter, her class-mates and teacher are walking around hand-in-hand in time to Moroccan music. The teacher is a woman of about thirty-five. She is not particularly pretty, but she is attractive. She has a nicely cut bob, she is thin and very smiley. What strikes me is how stylish she is. She wouldn't look out of place in the smart Place Vendôme in Paris. She is wearing a pair of jeans, a red and blue top and a wool scarf. She is doing something that would make most adults look ridiculous, stomping around in circles with a group of nursery-aged children. But she looks supremely elegant. How does she pull this off? Is it because she's French?

There's no denying French women do have a certain something. Anglo-Saxons have always admired the French sense of style. Even English soldiers during the Hundred Years' War were impressed with the French women and the way they looked. If your best friend tells you her husband has a Bulgarian mistress, you can at least console her and give her some hope. If she tells you he has a French mistress, you know your friend is toast. We can't compete with the French. Even Kate Moss can't compete with them; she lost out to Vanessa Paradis in the battle for Johnny Depp.

'Take an English woman and a French woman,' says Nadine, an English lawyer friend who lives in Paris. 'Give them both a pair of identical jeans, a white T-shirt and a pair of loafers and ask them to put them on. For some inexplicable reason the French woman will manage to carry off the outfit better and look more attractive.'

Style and design guru Anouska Hempel tells me this ability to look good is in fact arrogance. French women may be chic but they are sadly lacking in that most essential of qualities: a sense of humour. 'They have the impression that they are the most elegant and stylish people in the world,' she says. 'I think French women have being beautiful absolutely born into them. They think they're beautiful even when they're not, so they have a sort of extraordinary arrogance which exudes a rather strange sort of confidence that is often misplaced. We Anglo-Saxons come with a lot more humility, a lot more fun and a lot more humour.'

What is the truth? Maybe the French female arrogance has something to do with the way women have been revered in France. Even the symbol of France is a woman. Marianne, as she is called, is present in every town hall and every court of law. Her profile is engraved on coins, drawn on stamps and was on the banknotes until the introduction of the euro. Marianne became the official symbol of the Republic in 1792 but it wasn't until 1970 that she was modelled on a famous French woman. The sculptor Alain Aslan sculpted a bust of Brigitte Bardot. Since then models for Marianne have included Catherine Deneuve, Inès de la Fressange, Sophie Marceau and Laetitia Casta. A more impressive list of elegant and beautiful women would be difficult to find. But is their beauty anything to do with the fact that they're French?

Are French women innately elegant or just arrogant? Is the French beauty myth just that? A myth that they have perpetuated and we all believe because they invented *haute couture* and know how to tie a scarf? Or is their style a bit like their wine; once dominant, but now losing out to the new world? The major designers in Paris are now foreigners. French food, revered for centuries, has been overtaken by Italian, Chinese or even Thai cuisine. Some serious research is needed.

The best person to ask about style is an 'It' girl. That's because they really don't do much apart from being stylish, so they have to know more about it than the rest of us. France has only one 'It' girl. She is called Hermine de Clermont-Tonnerre and is famous for being, well, her. As is typical in egalitarian France, she comes from one of the most aristocratic and famous families in the country.

We arrange to meet on the exclusive Avenue Montaigne in Paris, home to all the major designers. I get there early and stand outside the restaurant she has designated as our meeting spot. I am bursting with curiosity to see what an 'It' girl looks like in real life. The only thing I have to go on after googling her and finding nothing at all is the fact that I have been told she might well have purple hair. So here I am on a drizzly morning, waiting for someone with strange coloured hair outside a posh restaurant in central Paris.

At the arranged time of our meeting I call her mobile phone to see if I'm in the right place. I see a very chic-looking girl across the street take her phone out of her bag and look at it. Could this be her? The girl doesn't have purple hair, but she has a Gucci bag, definitely an 'It' girl accessory. So why isn't she answering my call? The girl walks past me into the restaurant without so much as a second glance. Meanwhile another very trendy-looking girl drives by in a jet-black Smart car. She is obviously looking for somewhere to park. Maybe that's her? I phone again, it's now ten past ten. This time she picks up. I tell her I'm standing outside the restaurant.

'I'm there too,' says Hermine de Clermont-Tonnerre in English, but with a very seductive French accent.

'Where?' I look all around but can't see anyone.

'I see you,' she says.

'I can't see you, where are you?'

'Here,' announces France's answer to Paris Hilton, stepping out of a chauffeur-driven black Mercedes with black-tinted windows. A Smart car? Oh please. What was I thinking?

I now also know what she means when she told me I would recognise her. I have never seen anyone like her before. She is dressed in the most colourful outfit I have ever seen. And her hair actually matches it. Yes, there is some purple in there, but also green, red, yellow and blue. Oddly enough it doesn't look deranged. In fact I think she's rather beautiful, although I can imagine the French establishment finds her a little eccentric.

Her dress is by Dior. I only know that because her handbag has a big D on it and is made of the same material. It is one of those gypsy-like feminine, flowing dresses with a low front and lots of ruffles. She wears an Indian-style jacket, suede with beading all over it. I'm sure it's Gucci or something similar. Her skin is flawless and tanned, her eyes wide and clear. She wears a little shimmering lip gloss and mascara. Her nails are long and red and her eyebrows plucked into a dramatic arch. She is pregnant and looks great.

One of Hermine's hobbies is rally-driving and as she can't drive while pregnant she has just been officiating the start of a race. When she's not driving cars, she is riding her motorbike (all 1400 cc) around Paris. She tells me she is in the process of suing the police who recently stopped her, strip-searched her and threw her in a cell for six hours for having a motorbike that is too loud. I get the impression Hermine is not your run-of-the-mill French aristo.

On the question of French style she is rebellious. 'Oh it's so heavy here,' she says. 'People ask me why can't I wear black like everyone else, why do I have colour in my hair, why can't I be more like my mother? You English are much more fun, it's so much more normal to be original there.'

So is she telling me I have to stay English in order to be stylish? This would be a first.

'No, of course not,' she says. 'I think the French have an innate style, but maybe less than before. But I love the English, you're so crazy and funny. Although I don't think they can mix colours and styles as well as the French; but they are at least full of ideas.'

Hermine is married to a Scottish man called Alistair so

she has had plenty of exposure to Brits. She says that the one thing that really shocks her about English women is how drunk they get. 'French women are definitely more stylish when it comes to drinking,' she says. 'An English girl will drink and drink until she is drunk; it's horrible. I actually saw a woman vomit outside a restaurant in London last time I was there.'

I have an English friend called James who lives in Paris. He agrees with Hermine. 'If you walk into a room with a French girl, an English girl and an American girl, you can easily tell which is which,' he says. 'The French girl will greet you with a kiss, the English girl will be half-drunk and the American will be wearing some hoop earrings and bright colours.' James says that if he ever gives up on single life and marries, it won't be to an English girl. 'All they want to do is drink four cans of lager while watching the footie,' he says. 'I have mates who I can do that with, I don't need a ladette.'

Hermine finds the British much more open than the French, but says it is not always stylish. 'We are a little uptight, we don't talk about sex, religion or money here but for the British there are no limits. They talk about sex openly, anything. I like the eccentricity but I think it can be more seductive to have a little mystery.'

So French style is all about staying sober and secretive? Henri, a French friend of mine who now lives in London, says he is shocked by the way English women behave and dress. He says that whereas in France you might see a well-dressed woman with a bra strap showing, in England they go out wearing practically nothing but their underwear. 'They are drunk, vulgar and forward,' he says. 'When I first moved here, I realised all I needed to do to sleep with a girl was to ask her. But your culture is so different, maybe the only way they can get men to notice them is to be over the top.'

When I go back to England, the difference in the way the women dress is obvious. I've discovered I no longer dress in the same way I used to at home. I would never wear a mini-skirt now and it's not a conscious decision I've taken.

Something has come over me, some kind of French osmosis, while I wasn't paying attention. It may also of course be an age thing. A young girl in a mini-skirt can look great. What is worrying is someone over thirty five trying to look sexy by flaunting something she hasn't got. I have learnt some French restraint since moving here.

It's true what the French say—some English and American women have terrible dress sense. They are totally unaware of how to be sexy and stylish. Sexiness, as any French woman will tell you, is not about revealing everything. 'When the English go out, they dress up to the nines, to the point of being ridiculous,' says Dorothée Werner, a journalist with *Elle Magazine* in Paris. 'It's minus three degrees outside and you see all these girls wandering around half naked. A French girl would never do that; they don't want to give the impression that they've made a great effort. The ultimate chic is an old top and a pair of jeans.' This is getting confusing. Whatever happened to Chanel suits and strings of pearls?

I go along to meet Inès de la Fressange, the world's first supermodel. Before the meeting I am terrified. I spend an age deciding what to wear; I don't want to look too scruffy or too done up. I am intrigued to see what she will be wearing. I imagine her in some specially-designed Karl Lagerfeld creation.

She comes out smiling and kisses me warmly. She is about a foot taller than me and lovely. There really is no other word for it, Inès is stunning. And she's wearing a pair of jeans and an old sweater. We go to her office and she lights up one of about five cigarettes she will smoke during our hour and a half chat (OK, nobody's totally perfect). She makes me feel completely at home. This is someone who is so relaxed and charming you can't fail to like her, even if you're dying not to.

She tells me that she once got so sick of all the talk about fashion and style that she went to a party dressed in a pair of pyjamas. 'I had a tartan cashmere Hermès shawl on as well,' she says. 'Which was very chic. And of course the pyjamas were ironed and silk, but the fact remains that I was in pyjamas and nobody noticed. I think people get a little obsessed with how they dress and really no one cares that much.'

During the meeting her glass-topped coffee table crashes to the floor. Amazingly our coffees are still in their cups. 'Never buy anything from a junk shop,' she says laughing.

Inès tells me about one of her trips for Chanel to London. 'I was there to do what they call personal appearances, hand out perfume samples and meet people. I just had my Chanel case with me, full of my Chanel working clothes. Then my husband Luigi said we had been invited to stay with some friends for the weekend. I felt so bad, all I had to wear were my Chanel suits while everyone else was in jeans and wellies and so casual. They all kept saying to me 'oh that must have been *awfully* expensive' and I felt like an idiot.'

French women hate to be badly dressed, and by badly dressed they don't just mean in bad taste but in the wrong outfit for the event. The actress Elisabeth Bourgine, who famously wore nothing in the film *Cours Privé,* says the thing about French women is that they're adaptable. 'We can like classical music and rap, we can dress in an evening dress or like a rapper, but we would never confuse the two evenings,' she says.

The one thing a French woman will never wear in the wrong place is a pair of sneakers. In fact they will not wear sneakers unless they are engaging in some sporting activity. They can't even begin to understand the American habit of wearing sneakers to the office and then changing once you get there. Apart from anything else, it is just too much effort.

After my meeting with Inès, I take a taxi to meet the former justice minister and MP Elisabeth Guigou in her office at the *Assemblée Nationale*, the French equivalent of the House of Commons. I ask the taxi driver what the main difference is between French and foreign women. 'Sneakers,' he tells me 'The Americans are incapable of putting on a pair of shoes.'

Elisabeth Guigou is very beautiful and impeccably turned out, she has blonde hair, lovely blue eyes and beautiful skin. Her nails are manicured and painted an oyster white. She is wearing a suit. I am, however, shocked to see her wearing a pair of sneakers. This is first time I have ever seen a French woman in tennis shoes outside a tennis court. What on earth is going on? How can one of France's most illustrious politicians be breaking the first rule of female Frenchness? I conduct the interview and try to take my mind off the shoes. She is eloquent (speaks perfect English) and charming. She tells me that being a politician came relatively late to her. She was invited to join the government by Mitterrand (maybe he liked sneakers?) and it took her twenty-four hours to make the decision to accept his offer.

'I knew my life would never be the same again,' she says. 'I knew I would be working every weekend. There is so much work you wouldn't believe it.' Guigou tells me she relaxes by listening to music, being with her husband and son, reading and gardening. She has a particular passion for English roses. As she gets up to see me out, I notice she is limping. 'I broke my ankle,' she tells me. 'This is why I have to wear these.' She looks disdainfully at her shoes. I breathe a sigh of relief.

I ask every single French woman I meet if they ever wear sneakers other than when they are jogging or playing some kind of sport. For example Sylvie Tellier, who was Miss France two years ago, says she would never wear them outside the house, even to buy a loaf of bread. 'I might meet someone I know,' she tells me. I am tempted to ask her if this person would then wander around Paris in acceptable shoes blackening her reputation. Or maybe she would be thrown into jail. Is Paris crawling with state-sponsored style police?

These women are so annoyingly perfect I am suddenly longing to see a broken nail or a hair out of place. Don't they ever relax? Is it possible to be so blooming together all the time? How about downing half a bottle of Chardonnay and telling lewd jokes like we do back home?

One of the most perfect women in Paris is Agnès Cromback, CEO of Tiffany's. I go to meet her one day shortly after Easter. She is looking stunning in a dark suit and diaphanous shirt. Rather incongruously she is roaring with laughter at an electronic Easter card which features bunnies rapping to a tune she is totally taken with. 'What is this?' she asks me as I sit down. 'I have to get it, it's great.' It sounds familiar, but rap tunes are not my forte so I can't help her. But this is clearly a very elegant woman who has a sense of fun. I ask the million-dollar question.

'Would you ever wear a tracksuit and a pair of running shoes?'

'Of course,' she responds. I smile broadly, so they're not all as perfect as they make out. 'Every Sunday,' she continues. 'I wear a very nice tracksuit, all in white, and I go jogging. Then I come back and have a shower and get changed.'

'But would it ever occur to you to maybe stay in the tracksuit? It is Sunday, after all.'

Agnès looks horrified. 'Oh no, I couldn't do that. I know some people do, but to me it's like letting yourself go, as bad as getting fat.' Heaven forbid.

I ask Agnès if she dresses down when she gets home from the office. 'Yes, of course,' she replies. 'I take off my suit and jewellery and put on a nice cashmere top and trousers.' So really relaxed then. Agnès says we Anglo-

Saxons have little idea of how to dress down. 'I once saw one of my American bosses looking casual,' she says. 'He arrived carrying a backpack. He immediately lost all the authority he had.'

This ability to stay chic even when relaxing is one of the first rules of French style. It seems the men demand it. 'When I come back home from work, I don't want my wife wearing an old tracksuit and no make-up,' says Nicolas, a French male friend of mine. 'She can dress down, but not slob out.' Marie Sauvage, a very pretty blond girl who works in PR, says her husband comes home very late at night so she is ready for bed by the time he sees her. I ask her what she is wearing when he gets home, surely not make-up and a Chanel suit?

'Pyjamas,' she purrs. 'But very superior pyjamas.'

One important French style rule is to make an effort at all times and not skimp on the details. This means wearing good (read expensive) shoes, having the right earrings, necklace, scarf and so on to go with whatever you're wearing. You can be wearing an unremarkable outfit but if you accessorise it properly it can be turned into something else. Making an effort at all times includes your hair, nails, make-up and overall look. There are probably just as many plain girls in France as there are in England and America but they don't look plain.

They will invariably be thinner than the English girl. According to European Union statistics French women are the slimmest in Europe, weighing an average of 126 pounds, seven pounds less than British women. They will also know how to wear their hair and clothes and how to carry themselves. They walk properly, which I suppose might be partly down to that famous French arrogance.

In England we have Trinny and Susannah telling the nation how to dress. In France, there is no equivalent. I don't think I know a French woman who would put up with being told what to wear by a TV celebrity. Also French women have the whole of society dictating the way they dress, starting with their mothers and their cultural heritage. 'I don't think style is innate,' says my best French friend Alexandra. 'But if you have a stylish mother then you will copy her.' Sophie Tellier says it is a question of education. 'We live in an environment where you learn not to wear red with orange or squares with stripes,' she says.

Isabelle Hervé-Penard, the personal shopper at France's most prestigious department store, Galeries Lafayette in Paris, says that this confidence can sometimes be misplaced. 'French women are more confident about how to dress than other women,' says Isabelle who has clients from all over the world. 'They are confident because they are French. They have the history of fashion behind them so they think they know how to dress. They are not always right, so you have to guide them towards something else.'

Sabbia Rosa, who owns an exclusive underwear shop in Paris, agrees the French sense of style is part of their culture.

'It is something deep in her psyche,' she says. 'But it can also be constraining. For example we can't dress in the anarchic way the English or the Japanese do, we have the image of Coco Chanel in our head and we can't fight that.'

The funny thing is that as an English girl living here you find it increasingly hard to fight as well. Jeanette Franklin, originally from Yorkshire, has been living in France for nearly fifteen years. We meet for a drink in the Irish pub in Montpellier. I ask her if she has changed since she moved here. 'Totally,' she says. 'I used to have brown hair, now I'm blonde, I didn't wear make-up, now I wear it all the time, I didn't wax, now I do, I used to have great big bushy eyebrows, now I have thin ones, I used to wear grey faded underwear, now it's all matching and sparkling.'

Jeanette works at the French-American centre in Montpellier and she sees this transformation in the students that come there as well. 'They arrive looking grungy and leave looking sexy,' she says. 'As an English girl if you walk around Montpellier for half a day you start to feel dowdy and want to change.'

Having lived here for five years, I believe French women do have a certain something. And not only do I want to know what it is, but I want some of it. I too want to look effortlessly elegant in a pair of jeans and white T-shirt with my hair tied loosely back. I too want to be able to walk in a room and not be immediately recognised as an English woman before I even open my mouth. I want this indefinable and alluring chic that French women have. But I don't want to lose my sense of humour along with my green wellies and boob tube. It seems I will have to proceed with care.

2

Zen Exercise

'I'm French, so I'm quite lazy about exercising, and I smoke.
But I do love going for a run in the morning with my dog.
That's all.'
Eva Green

Before we moved to France, I had been going to gyms
for years. I hated it, of course, but couldn't see any
other way to stay in shape. I would go to step classes.
A more disheartening way of spending a Saturday morning
is hard to imagine. A vicious woman dressed in pink with a
microphone attached to her sweatband would be shrieking
'step' and 'grapevine' at the top of her voice as I would
stumble around trying to coordinate my body. Multi-
tasking I can do: I can interview someone for an article,

while feeding a baby, cooking dinner and putting the washing machine on. But ask me to move my arms and legs in opposing though coordinated directions at the same time and I freeze.

We have been living in France for a couple of months when I meet Beatrice. You'd think with a name like that she would be French. Not a bit of it. She is married to a Frenchman but extremely English. Which is lucky as when I meet her at a lunch party I speak hardly a word of French and have been panicking all week about how long I can stretch my French (limited to what's your name and where do you live) over what is bound to be a four-course feast.

Beatrice and I get chatting; she tells me how she's lived in France for over twenty years, how she met her French husband Luc and ended up in one of the region's most splendid houses. She looks extremely French; impeccably turned out, beautiful, and pencil thin. I have just given birth and am keen to lose the excess weight I have gained during pregnancy. I ask Beatrice what she does to stay fit.

She tells me all about a gym class she goes to, run by a local lady called Madame Clerc. She says it is at 8 o'clock in the morning on Tuesdays and Fridays and suggests I go with her. The 8 o'clock kick-off sounds terrible, but when she explains that it is just a bit of stretching I figure I can manage that without any trouble at all. After all, seven years on, I have finally mastered the 'grapevine.' What could be worse than that? I don't think for a moment some little gym class in the middle of southern France will pose any serious threat to this seasoned London gym-goer.

At ten minutes past eight that first Tuesday, I am sweating, red-faced and practically unable to breathe. Madame Clerc's class may be about stretching, but it is the most physically exhausting thing I have ever done (and I include childbirth in that). We are asked to contort our bodies into various positions on the floor. Essentially it is a question of using your body weight as resistance. The movements are graceful and slow, almost like a dance, we do three routines of about seven minutes each (not that I'm counting) before moving to the bar and mat work. At the bar we stretch and bend and do countless *pliés*. My thighs feel like they are on fire. There are times I wanted to scream 'mercy' at the top of my voice, but the serene faces of the other participants (all, apart from Beatrice, a good twenty years my senior) stop me. On the mat Madame Clerc talks us through a sit-up regime that would have had Steve Redgrave weeping.

But the extraordinary thing about it all is that the movements are all extremely fluid and must look effortless, if you ignore my puce-red face. Madame Clerc ends with what I call stretches, and she calls cooling down. Her favourite is one whereby you bend down to hold your ankles and then bend and straighten your knees several times, increasing the stretch with each one. This she tells us we must do every day, with our legs together and also shoulder-width apart. She tells us if we ever bend down to pick something up, to do it with straight legs. Every stretch counts is Madame Clerc's motto.

Once I am able to walk again, about two days after the first class, I go to lunch with Sylvie, a French friend from Montpellier. She has had four children but doesn't seem to have an ounce of fat on her. I ask her about her fitness regime. She laughs and says she has never been to a gym in her life. 'I just move,' she tells me. 'If it's a choice between the stairs and a lift, I take the stairs. I get up earlier in the morning so I can cycle to work instead of driving. Moving is part of my everyday life.'

Later that week I interview a famous French politician called Clara Gaymard. Clara is Head of the French Inward Investment Agency, so responsible for attracting foreign investment to the country. She and her husband Hervé, who was France's Finance Minister until revelations that the state was paying about ten thousand pounds a month for his luxury flat in Paris forced him to resign, have had eight children. Can you imagine? And yes, you guessed it: she is pencil thin and scarily elegant. How does she do it? 'I don't ever exercise,' she tells me. 'But I do a lot of running around; with eight children you have no choice.' A friend of mine informs me that Madame Gaymard also has five staff to help her, which is about five more than the average mother of eight has.

But I now understand that the way French women

exercise is completely different from the way we do. They don't really go for bouncing around. They do move, but they don't believe in sweating a lot. They go for a more serene form of exercise which is more elegant and, well, French.

The women I speak to who do formal exercise tend to do it in the privacy of their own home with a personal trainer. 'Exercise, like dieting, should be done in solitude,' says one. The other big difference is that they don't do weights. To a French woman, the idea of building up muscles so you look sinewy is anathema. At a party I went to in London recently, there were several women of an indefinable age with great big shoulders and arms. They looked positively scary and it's not a look the French would find either acceptable or attractive.

French women have some extraordinary role models when it comes to exercise. The French novelist Colette called exercise 'physical culture' and saw it as integral part to her intellectual well-being as well as her physical state. She would travel with her mobile gym, a contraption made up of two wooden bars which she would contort herself over in various positions. This is a woman who was still dancing half-naked on tables aged over sixty. An inspiration to us all, and if you follow my advice, you don't even need the mobile gym. Diane de Poitiers (1490-1566), Henri II's mistress, started each day with a cold bath at 6 o'clock in the morning and then went for a three-hour horseback ride and kept her slender figure until she died.

French women don't go for binge-exercising either, which is what I used to do at home. I would go to the gym once a week and sweat like a lunatic and then do nothing else for the next six days but drink and eat. They treat exercise rather like they do food; a little every day. Most of the French women I know say they don't do any particular form of formal exercise, maybe one or two yoga classes, but they all say they move.

For example, they walk every day. Inès de la Fressange is the quintessential French woman in that respect. She says the secret to her slim silhouette is shopping. 'If you shop a lot, you walk for miles and stay thin,' she says. I have to agree with her. Two days in Paris and the weight falls off me, despite all the good things I eat when I'm there. Just walking around one of the French department stores is the equivalent of a three-mile hike. And then there's all the effort of taking your clothes off and putting them on again to try others on. Exhausting, I reckon it's possible to burn at least two hundred calories an hour, as well as two hundred pounds.

James, my English friend who has lived in Paris for almost ten years, argues that French women don't so much have a philosophy on exercise, rather they just don't like it. 'They want as much result as possible for as little effort,' he says. 'So they will do things like walking and tennis and so on because it doesn't seem like hard work. They hate the idea of sweating over weights. The other thing they do a lot is sex. I sometimes think they see that as a form of keeping fit. They are quite tough to get into bed, but once you've got them there it's morning, noon and night.'

Yvette, a thirty-something woman I met in Paris while researching this book, says she uses her lovers as just that; a workout. 'Men have been abusing women for decades, so why not treat them as objects for once? I refuse to go to a gym and as I live close to the office can easily nip home for a rendezvous,' she says. 'I am as fit as I was in my twenties and much happier. It's also cheaper than the gym so I can spend the money I save on sexy underwear and make-up.' I have to admit; when I met her for a coffee in a classy little café opposite the Louvre she looked great, full of confidence and fun. I wondered whether she had just come from a work-out, or whether she was on her way to one.

Sylvie, my Montpellier friend, says she has a friend who uses her husband as a workout. 'He is mad about sex,' she tells me. 'She's not. So what she does is treat it like a workout, she goes on top most of the time, and focuses on working out her thighs while holding in her stomach muscles. He's happy as anything and has no clue he is an alternative to a gym class.'

Florence Pernel, an extremely pretty, successful TV actress here, tipped to become the French equivalent of Helen Mirren, agrees traditional exercise methods are not for the French. 'Essentially we French women like a nice way of life and that doesn't include gyms and spending hours doing sit-ups. We are lazy and like the maximum effect for the least effort. We have creams that can do all the hard work.'

French women spend more than 91 million dollars a year on slimming creams and gels. I never believed in them until I moved here. But research carried out by the French National Institute for Consumer Protection shows they can make a difference. They tested ten brands on two hundred women and found that volunteers lost up to two centimetres around their thighs in fourteen days.*

Some French women, such as the actress Elisabeth Bourgine, prefer to cycle. She says she stays thin that way. As cycling is a national obsession, almost as popular as having affairs, I feel I have to try it. I can't really say I have integrated if I haven't been on a bike.

I start with a mountain bike and cycle around the vineyards. It is great for my thighs and buttocks and a brilliant way to walk the dogs. My husband has by this stage bought himself a racing bike and has become totally obsessed with the whole thing. He even watches the Tour de France and reads *Vélo Magazine*. He goes out three times a week with a gang of retirees from the village. At least that is what he says he does. He leaves the house at 7.40 in the morning wearing skin-tight lycra and comes back at

---

* The two top-scoring creams were L'Oréal's Plénitude Perfect Slim and Elancyl's Concentré-Lissant Chrono-Actif.

midday, sweating and panting. He certainly seems a lot fitter.

He suggests I get into road biking as well. 'You can see so much more. Go so much further,' he tells me. 'Here, have my old bike. I need a new one.' He presents me with a black racing bike with those funny pedals you need special clip-in shoes for.

I knew it was a bad idea the minute I got on. At the bottom of our drive I try to stop and unclip my shoe. Of course the thing won't come out and all I can do is wail as I slowly topple over, grazing the whole side of my body.

My husband, who thinks people falling over is incredibly funny, almost falls off his bike as well, he is laughing so much.

The next time we go out we cycle over to lunch at some friends'. When I arrive, thinking I have mastered the shoe thing, I joke: 'Wouldn't it be un-cool to fall over on their doorstep as they open the door instead of getting off the bike looking serene in my lycra kit?' That's exactly what happens, and so some of Paris's most stylish people look on horrified as the black bike and I collapse in front of them.

The third and final time we ever go cycling together is to buy the Sunday papers in a nearby village. They get the *Sunday Times* delivered on a Sunday and as it is about five miles away it seems like a nice idea to cycle there in the spring sunshine. We get the paper. I am so completely engrossed in an article about thongs being last week's look that I forget that starting on an incline with both feet clipped in is not a good idea. I get about one inch, then the bike stops and I just know what is coming next. I try in vain to throw the paper on the ground to cushion the blow with its size. I think I've broken my arm (for about a minute) and decide never to get on the thing again. Much as I love amusing my husband, there have to be other, less painful ways to do so.

Despite this early setback, my transformation into a French exerciser goes on. I go for at least three walks a day. One of them is up a ferocious hill, which I go up and down four times when I have enough time. Every morning when I wake up, I do fifty sit-ups, thirty-five push-ups and fifty bottom clenches; but all *à la française*, none of the body-building jerking movements I used to endure in London gyms. The whole approach is somehow more Zen.

To do the sit-ups (which I learnt in Madame Clerc's class but also saw on the back of a cereal packet here, so I am guessing they are universally approved by French women and experts and therefore infallible), you lie on your back but raise your body onto your elbows. You then lift both legs in the air (holding your stomach in if it's physically possible) and lower them slowly to the ground. Then bring them back up again. Repeat this twenty five times. For the next set you start in the same position but lift and lower alternate legs. This one is easier, if you find it too easy then lie down. The push-ups are done against a wall, not on the floor. You stand about two feet from the wall with your hands flat against it. You then bounce yourself back to an upright position, using your arms. Then go back to the starting position by letting yourself fall towards the wall with your hands out in front of you. Repeat this thirty five times. The buttock clenches consist of lying down and lifting your haunches in the air, your shoulders and feet are on the ground. You lift and clench twenty five times. The second set is smaller lifts and clenches; you basically stay higher up and repeat the reduced movement twenty five times.

Buttock clenches can be done at any stage during the day, as can stomach exercises. I just hold my stomach in whenever I think about it; I soon started to notice a difference. Pelvic floor muscles are a really good thing to exercise whenever you're bored. If I'm at a dinner sitting next to someone who insists on discussing commuting or childcare, I find it an ideal opportunity to improve my pelvic floor. It's got to the stage now that when we leave a dinner my husband will not ask if I had a good time, but rather: 'How's your pelvic floor?'

You might think there isn't enough time to do all this walking and squeezing. The little sit-up/push-up/buttock clenching routine takes all of ten minutes. The hill walking I do in the morning before the children go to school, usually with the boy in the pram, thus enhancing the work-out, and the pelvic floor training, well, you can do them while you're reading this. I also try to go for a walk at night after dinner.

The French method is to look on any opportunity to move as one not to be missed. There is no need to compartmentalise your day into a time for exercising and a time for not exercising; be aware of the opportunities you have during the day to improve your fitness and take them. As Sylvie says: 'If you think about the way your body looks and are aware of it, then you will work harder to improve it. Why only think about it for an hour a week?'

Madame Clerc's philosophy was the same. 'Think about stretching all the time, it is the most essential thing,' she would say as she bent over and effortlessly placed her flat palms on the floor. She really was the most inspiring teacher I ever had. Tragically she was killed a couple of years ago while out cycling with her husband.

Since I moved here, I do think about my body a lot more. This is one of the ways in which I have become more French. I think about standing up tall and sitting up straight, I think about holding my stomach in and clenching my buttocks whenever I have the chance. I am much more aware of the way I walk and hold myself. My attitude to exercise now is more fundamental, a part of everyday life. If the children want to go for a walk, I see it as an opportunity to move, if they want to play in the garden, I do some Madame Clerc stretches or lunges while I watch them. If I'm stuck in a traffic jam, I pull in my stomach and squeeze my pelvic floor. I even look forward to helping my husband move the piles of logs we store for winter, though of course I wear rubber gloves so as not to damage my nails. The result is a firmer body and a clear conscience. There's nothing worse than that irritating voice in your head saying 'I must do some exercise' over and over again. Nowadays I rarely hear it.

3

The Secret Weapon

'Being naked is a declaration of an intention.
Wearing suspenders is a secret.'
French Anonymous

I get on the 7.49 TGV at Béziers to Paris. I am in a
window seat. The children had been waking me up all
night so I quickly fall asleep. I register at Montpellier
that someone comes and sits next to me but fall asleep
again and wake up an hour or so later. I study my
neighbour. From what I can see, he is very good-looking
in a distinguished sort of way. He is wearing a dark blue
suit with a pale pink shirt and tie. He has brown hair,
streaked with grey. He is reading an extremely intellectual looking book. I pretend to stretch and look around the

carriage so I can get a better look at him.

'Did you sleep well?' he asks. His accent is not regional, he is obviously from Paris. 'Yes, thank you, I needed to catch up' I reply. He smiles.

'Where are you from?' When I tell him, he immediately closes his book. He was at Oxford University, he tells me in flawless, if gorgeously accented, English. He adores England, where he spent some of the happiest days of his life. We spend the rest of the journey talking. B, as I will call him, tells me he is an MP and on his way to the *Assemblée Nationale*. He reminds me of a well-built Dominique de Villepin, the handsome French Prime Minister who is tipped as one of Chirac's possible successors. B tells me has been on business in Montpellier but lives mainly in Paris and sometimes on his family's estate in Burgundy. He asks me what I do and why I am going to Paris.

'I'm going to write about French women and lingerie,' I tell him.

'And is this a subject of which you know much?'

'Not yet,' I reply, feeling slightly embarrassed. 'But I'm hoping to learn.'

B laughs and tells me the most important thing to understand about women and their lingerie is that they wear it for themselves and not for men. He drops me off in a taxi at my hotel in Saint-Germain. We exchange cards.

'*J'ai été ravi d'avoir fait votre connaissance,*' he says when we part.

'Call me if you ever need anything in Paris.' He kisses my hand and gets back in the taxi.

I have work to do and begin at Galeries Lafayette in Paris. A mecca dedicated to French female pleasure, this is where France's wealthy, famous and glamorous women have shopped since 1893. Its ten floors have everything a woman could possibly want, including ten thousand square feet dedicated to bras, panties and corsets.

It is impossible to know where to start. There is everything you could want; from La Perla and Dior to Calvin Klein and Princesse Tam-Tam. I wander around in a daze for about half an hour, wondering how you would ever choose anything. Finally I decide to start interviewing people.

Amazingly the first person I accost is English. She is as stunned as I am by the choice on offer. 'It's unbelievable,' says Samantha from Hull, who is in Paris for a two-day break and shopping for underwear. 'I used to work at Selfridge's and we had about a third as much space dedicated to underwear, which just goes to show that French women demand more choice than we do.'

Historically the French have always been ahead of the British and Americans in terms of underwear. They were wearing knickers way before us. In around 1530 Queen Catherine de Medici introduced them as she preferred to ride side-saddle to show off her legs and needed to protect herself from the elements. The Brits still thought panties scandalous and only fit to be worn by prostitutes. In 1663 Samuel Pepys wrote in his diary that the wearing of knickers by his French wife was a sure sign of infidelity.

Panties weren't really accepted until the nineteenth century when the Victorian guardians of morality and health seized upon them as a good thing. 'Drawers are of incalculable advantage to women who expose themselves to a variety of diseases from the unusual form of their garments,' states the 1841 *Handbook of the Toilet*, a must-read for any self-respecting Victorian. 'In France, drawers form a necessary part of female attire, and many indispositions to which British females are continually subject are prevented by their use.'

The *brassière*, derived from the French word for upper arm, or bra, first appeared in France at the turn of the century. Prior to this women had worn corsets. The arrival of the bra meant they were liberated from this imprisoning garment which made moving and even breathing difficult. It was invented by Herminie Cadolle (1845-1926), founder of the Cadolle lingerie house. In 1889 she opened a lingerie workshop where she invented a two-piece garment, a lower part for the waist and an upper part supporting the breasts which was called a *soutien-gorge* (breast support) a name that is still used today in France. Herminie exhibited her bra at the 1900 Great Exposition and became a fitter of bras to the elite of the day, including Mata Hari.

I speak to some other shoppers and ask them what they

look for when they buy underwear. 'I buy nice underwear in order to look sexy when I take my clothes off,' says Claire, an elegant forty-two-year-old Parisian woman. 'It's fundamental for me,' Nathalie, aged thirty eight, also from Paris, tells me. 'It's the first thing I put on so it determines my whole mood.' Some French women say that underwear is so essential because it is so intimate. 'It's what I put on next to my skin, so it has to be perfect,' says Julie, twenty eight, from Amiens.

After the interviews I decide it is important for my continued research to try some underwear. The changing rooms at Galeries Lafayette are sumptuous, beautifully decorated in pink. There are two buttons on the wall; one summons an assistant to help you with sizes and styles. The other changes the light inside the cubicle from day to night, so you can see at the flick of a switch how your new bra will look when your lover undresses you. I spend at least two happy hours flicking the switch on and off in several ensembles. I wonder briefly what B's tastes in underwear are, probably something subtle and sophisticated. Then it's back to work.

I visit the doyenne of French lingerie, Chantal Thomass, in her extravagantly decorated apartment in Paris's exclusive sixth arrondissement. I first came across Chantal Thomass on a visit to Marseille where there was an exhibition celebrating her work. She is a striking figure, classically French with a sharply cut bob which she has had for years and which is also her logo. She always wears black, on top that is. Underneath, she tells me, she wears all manner of colours. Her lips are always perfectly coloured with bright red lipstick.

Her apartment is reminiscent of her underwear collections; lots of pink, yards of stunning fabrics and patterns. I sit on a vast cream sofa in her drawing room which has two full-length windows looking out on the road below and a chandelier hanging from the ceiling. It is the perfect setting to create expensive and exclusive underwear.

Chantal began her career as a designer but found that her models were lacking proper underwear to wear with her creations. So she started to design some and it quickly caught the attention of the press. 'I would show maybe two minutes of underwear during a show,' she says. 'And it was always that bit that got picked up, so I became known for that.'

Chantal tells me that British women actually buy more underwear than French women, but it's cheaper and more likely to be from Marks & Spencer. 'They don't have the same culture of sophisticated lingerie that we French have,' she says, lighting up another of about ten menthol cigarettes she smokes throughout our interview. 'Of course French women demand comfortable underwear, but it must also be pretty. In addition, their underwear must be well-designed, made from high-quality materials and enhance the way they feel about themselves. Lingerie is fundamental to the way a woman feels. If your underwear isn't right, nothing else works.'

This might sound ridiculous, but a lot of women I speak to on the subject agree.

Sylvie Tellier, for example, the former Miss France, says underwear is essential to her. 'For me, if you're a beautiful woman, you have to start with beautiful underwear,' she says, looking predictably stunning in the drawing room of her new apartment. 'If I start with a good base, then I know I will dress well as I can't put ugly things on top.' The actress Elisabeth Bourgine agrees. 'Underwear sets the whole tone for the day. If I want to seduce, I wear a certain ensemble, if I am filming and have to be comfortable, I wear another,' she says. One woman I met at a party recently told me she has a friend who has three hundred and sixty five sets of bras and panties; one for every day of the year. Now that's dedication. How would you choose which one to wear on any particular day? And where on earth does she keep them all? Does she have a special 'smalls' room where she spends many happy hours trying them all on?

Underwear is a lot more important to French women than it is to your average English girl, or at least this average English girl. Prior to moving to France it really wasn't an issue I had thought that much about. When I stayed with my father's friend Sophie all those years ago in the rue du Bac, she had the most amazing underwear. I was so keen to be like her I even bought a bra from a nearby shop. It's still too big. Sophie would wear garters, which I had never even seen before. I asked her what they were for. 'Garters are for seducing men,' she told me. Intrigued as I was by this concept, once I got home my interest in underwear faded. It was only now coming back again. Was this going to be my year in garters?

I decide that in order to gain a better understanding of my subject matter a visit to Chantal Thomass' shop on the rue Saint-Honoré is essential. The rue Saint-Honoré is in the most exclusive district of Paris, a continuation of the Faubourg Saint-Honoré where all the major *haute couture* houses are based. I immediately recognise her boutique as it is decorated a little like her apartment. A very pretty sales assistant asks me if she can help. I explain who I am and my quest for an insight into French women and their lingerie.

We wander around the shop and I pick out some underwear in pink and black gingham with lace. The minute I put it on I finally understand what all the fuss is about. The first time you try on a properly cut set of underwear, you understand how much it can do to enhance your body. I look totally different. The underwear I have been wearing seemed shabby and unstructured in comparison. My whole body takes on a more defined and sexier shape. This is incredible, I need to try some more.

Delphine, as the sales assistant is called, brings me in several things to try. It is such fun, like being given access to a pervy but classy dressing-up box. Maybe the lighting is cleverly arranged but I feel about twice as sexy as I have in years.

Among the most stunning examples is a leopard-print corset with g-string and stockings. I ask the sales girl if I'm not a little bit too old for this get-up. Delphine looks at me quizzically and says there are no age limits. I remember Chantal telling me that underwear has now become a fashion accessory, that you can wear it as clothes. 'For example, if you put on a corset with a pair of jeans and a shirt that you leave slightly open, you are dressed for anything,' she says.

I decide she is undoubtedly right and that a leopard-print corset (with garter belt of course) is an invaluable part of any girl's wardrobe. Delphine even says she'll throw in the leopard-print stockings for free. How can I resist such an offer?

I ask her how one washes these exquisite garments and my worst fears are confirmed when she tells me they have to be hand-washed. 'But just take them in the shower with you.' What could be easier?

According to Delphine, French women who live abroad often come home to Paris to stock up on underwear. 'They can't find the same elegance and sexiness away from Paris,' she tells me. 'They come here and bulk-buy before going back. You have to remember that for French women underwear is the key to their self confidence.' As I hand over almost the monthly average salary for three ensembles,

I wonder briefly who these rich French women bulk-buying might be.

I open the door to leave the shop and go to my next meeting, laden down with my gorgeously expensive Chantal Thomass pink shopping bags. As I wave goodbye to Delphine, about twenty Japanese women force their way in past me, giggling hysterically. They will probably spend more than the GDP of a small African country within minutes.

Next I visit Marie-Pierre Lannelongue, Fashion Editor of *Elle* in Paris. *Elle* is the one magazine that all French women concerned with fashion read. Aurélie, a friend of mine who is brand director for Chanel in Europe, calls it 'the bible.' According to Marie-Pierre underwear is playing an increasingly crucial role in a girl's wardrobe. 'The big thing now is the concept of over and under. That is you wear underwear that shows slightly, maybe a camisole or a g-string,' she tells me in the editor's office of the 'bible'. It is a fabulous room with vast glass windows and prior covers of the magazine acting as wallpaper. 'But this must never look like it's been done on purpose, it has to be subtle or it becomes vulgar. We are seeing an integration of underwear into women's wardrobes, it is no longer something that one just puts on underneath clothes, underwear are the new clothes.'

Some French women are willing to go out wearing only their underwear. I meet nineteen-year-old Parisian Nadine at Sabbia Rosa's exclusive lingerie shop looking for a *negligée* she is going to wear to a university ball in Cambridge. 'All those ball-gowns the English wear make me feel like I'm going to a fancy dress party,' she tells me. 'I couldn't possibly think of going out like that.' She chooses a scarlet silk *negligée* which looks great on her as she has a dark complexion and black hair. She also buys a flimsy silk wrap to go on top of it. I hope the weather in Cambridge will be clement on her big night.

Sabbia Rosa opened her boutique in Paris's sixth arrondissement in the 1960s. 'It was at the height of the feminist movement and people were burning their bras, not buying them,' she says. 'They would laugh as they walked past the shop, but I have always believed lingerie is fundamental to the French female psyche, and in the end I made it.'

Sabbia is one of the most charming and vivacious women you could ever meet. She is a grandmother but looks more glamorous than most teenagers with her incredible curly thick hair and cat-like green eyes. She is always impeccably turned out, often in her own underwear. When I meet her she is wearing one of her little slips with jeans and a cashmere cardigan and high heels.

'Life is tough for a woman nowadays and I think beautiful underwear gives her something nothing else can,' she says. 'Confidence and assurance. Even if they alone know that underneath the business suit lurks red silk, it is crucial to them.' Sabbia's prices are quite steep. A silk slip will set you back about a very substantial amount, and then of course you have to have the matching underwear. This is the one thing every single French woman I spoke to agreed on. Underwear must be matching. It is a fundamental and never to be broken rule. When I told Christine, a French friend of mine, that I was astounded by the fact that the French all wear matching underwear she said: 'Is there any other kind?'

French women don't mind spending money on underwear; in fact they budget for it as it is such an essential part of their wardrobe. A woman I met in Paris who has been a mistress for fifteen years says she spends ninety per cent of her salary on underwear. 'It's all very simple and always in beige, black or white,' she says. 'But I like expensive brands.' I can only assume her lover does too and so pays her rent.

Odile Morvan store director of underwear at Galeries Lafayette says underwear is all about seduction. 'But it may not be the seduction of someone else,' she tells me. 'For a French woman this can mean the seduction of herself, to feel good about herself and happy in her skin.'

Of course they also wear underwear to seduce, just like the rest of us. One of France's most popular celebrities, the actress and writer Anny Duperey says: 'When you see a secretary arrive at the office wearing stockings you just know she has not come just to do the accounts, it's not possible.' I saw a brilliant advertisement for lingerie recently in a French magazine. There was a picture of a woman dressed in a sexy corset, leaning seductively against a wall. 'He promised me fidelity,' reads the caption. 'I'll make the task easier.'

But according to Sébastien, a French male friend of mine who lives in London, one of the fundamental differences between French and English women is that when an English woman wants to be seductive, she will show her underwear. A French woman will not. 'It's so tacky,' he says. 'They will have a bra-strap showing really obviously, or their g-string riding up above their jeans. A French woman will of course also show a little, to give a hint, but this must never look forced or sluttish. It must look like it is an accident otherwise it's not attractive.'

My friend James tells me that another difference between French and English or American women is that French women love to unwind in sexy underwear. 'They're fantastically into it,' he says. 'You can be lying on the sofa on a Sunday morning, as hung-over as anything, and they start prancing around in the sexiest of outfits. An English girl would be there with her tracksuit bottoms and Gap hooded top.'

Everywhere you go in France, there are smart underwear shops, even in the small town where I live. I used to walk past thinking, why on earth would you bother spending $150 on a pair of panties and a bra. Now I wander past thinking, have I got time to try them on?

All You Need to Be Impossibly French

The transformation from an English underwear non-wearer to a French obsessive seems to have happened imperceptibly. When I first moved here, I would wear a pair of cotton underwear with whatever bra came to hand. Don't ask me how, but this has all changed now. I feel like I am part of a Stepford-wife-style conspiracy. Do they put something in the wine? Suddenly I find it impossible to break the rules, to wear non-matching underwear. I would as soon wear odd shoes. I am now always late going anywhere as it is essential I leave the house in matching underwear. So if I have decided on a bra that will go well under whatever outfit and I can't find the matching panties, I have to start all over again. I also spend more on a single set of underwear than I would have done in a whole year at home. An M&S five-pack is a thing of the past. What has happened to me? Will I ever be cured?

There is however one notable exception to the French mania for underwear. Inès de la Fressange. 'I only ever wear white cotton,' she says. 'To me all this lace is quite pathetic, it's just something women use to wake their husbands up when they have nothing else to offer. It's not for me. And I've been happily married for fourteen years.'

I leave Sabbia's shop and walk to my hotel which is in the same street. The receptionist tells me there is a card waiting for me and hands me a cream envelope. On the front is written in black ink Mme Frith Powell. I take it up to my room and sit on the bed. Inside is a postcard of a

Toulouse-Lautrec painting of a girl sitting half-naked on a floor, her stockings hanging loosely around her thighs. It reads: I hope you had a successful trip and I look forward to seeing the fruits of your research one day, Yours B.

I get back on the train later that evening after two days of deep immersion in underwear. Of course I am wearing my new Chantal Thomass underwear. Not the leopard-print ensemble which really would be a bit much for a train journey, but the pink gingham. You never know who you might run into on a train and, as every French woman knows, your underwear can make or break you.

4

Never Mind the Botox

'Age does not protect you from love. But love,
to some extent, protects you from age.'
Jeanne Moreau

If he is good enough for the TV star Anne Robinson, he is good enough for me. I make sure my husband is out before I make the call. His solution to his wife's ageing problems would be to trade her in for a younger model. Added to which he hates plastic surgery. It is a tough decision, but I figure this doesn't really count as surgery. And when it's all done he'll be happy he's married to someone with less wrinkles than the children.

I speak to a woman in London who says that the doctor

is extremely busy, but that he can fit me in three months from now. I will have to make up a reason for going to London.

'How much will it cost?' I ask, trying to sound casual about it.

'It works out at about $730 per wrinkle,' comes the reply.

Oh help, how many wrinkles do I have? Where should I stop? This bill could run into millions.

The next thing to get stressed about is any tell-tale signs that will give me away. Will there be any evidence that I had been 'botoxed'?

'There might be a bit of bruising,' said the voice. 'But it will pass in a few days.'

This is starting to sound uncomfortable.

Still, I make the appointment and tell my husband I am going to London to see my publisher. I feel like a woman with a lover, plotting her secret rendezvous. Sadly my date is with a man in a white coat and a needle filled with poison.

A couple of weeks after I make the appointment with the anti-wrinkle man my husband and I are invited to a book launch in London. It is a rather glittering event, full of famous people I fail to recognise like Princess Michael of Kent and Tim Rice. The odd thing is though, that apart from two good friends of mine, (one of whom when she spots me immediately drops the minor celebrity she is with saying 'Oh my God, there's another normal person, I have to go and speak to her') the women all look slightly odd.

Most of them are of an indeterminate age which could be anything from twenty five to fifty five. I know for a fact that Princess Michael of Kent is old enough to be my mother, but she looks like a spanking new Barbie doll that has just come off the production line. There are two other Barbie dolls standing talking to each other close to us. Their faces show no expression, they are so botoxed or pulled or whatever, that they look like blank slates. The only sign of life comes from their over-sized lips which look like they have been repeatedly punched. It's a little like walking into a horror movie.

Someone comes up and introduces herself. She is the mother of a friend of mine. The woman can hardly walk but has platinum blonde hair. Her face looks as if someone has put some cling-film over it and pulled it together at the back of her head as hard as they can. Her make-up is slightly smudged. The woman is clearly blind as well as rickety. Who does the think she is fooling in her sparkling shoes and trendy suit?

When we get back to Montpellier we go to a similarly glittering event, this time it is all French style. It is the launch of a new wine. There are lots of women there of all sorts of ages. The difference is that you can vaguely tell how old they are. Or at least if they're over forty. And they look a lot more elegant. They are dressed in colours that complement them, their hair is nicely done, some of them are even going a little grey, but they are not trying to compete with their grand-daughters. It is a big contrast with London.

French women do have plastic surgery. There are some notable examples, Isabelle Adjani and Emmanuelle Béart for example, two of the world's most beautiful women. One wonders what got into them. Béart now has that dazed fish look due to lip injections. Adjani has allegedly been having surgery since she was about twenty. Even one France's most gorgeous older actresses has had something done judging by the state of her ears; but she manages to carry it off due to her charisma and intelligence.

What is extraordinary is the young ones that are under the impression that if they have it done now, they will never have wrinkles. Hermine de Clermont-Tonnerre tells me the story of a friend of hers who works on *Le Monde* whose daughter, aged fifteen, demanded a breast enhancement for Christmas. Her mother naturally told her to forget about it. But it is terrifying that the girl even considered it.

One of the world's most famous plastic surgeons is French. He is called Dr Sebagh and divides his time between Paris and London where he has clinics. This is the man to see if you have an ageing problem. Or in fact any problem that can be remedied through botox or surgery.

The fact that he is French is perfect; I obviously need to speak to him to find out more about the French attitude to style. And he might even throw in the odd botox injection as a gesture of goodwill. Or better still tell me I have a rare type of non-ageing skin which only one in seven million are born with and so I have no need for him. I call his office and tell the receptionist who I am and what I am doing.

'Who?' barks the receptionist.

I explain who I am again.

'Weeeellll,' she drawls, Jeremy Paxman-like. 'You have to understand that Dr Sebagh is possibly THE busiest man in the WORLD.'

'Yes, of course,' I reply trying to sound suitably humble and impressed. 'He must be busier than God himself.'

'Why don't you send us an email and I'll talk to him.' I write an email and send it. Six months later I am still waiting for a reply.

French women don't seem to react to ageing quite as violently as we do. I think this is because they know that you can still be attractive when you're older. As the actress Anny Duperey, who is fifty-seven says: 'We might do some plastic surgery but we use it with caution and to take away something that is ungracious, not necessarily to trick people into thinking we're younger.' Elisabeth Bourgine agrees. 'To erase the passage of time is a mistake,' she says. 'The most beautiful thing in a face is expressions. It's better to have a few wrinkles than a face with no emotions.'

When I met Sabbia Rosa for the first time I found it hard to guess how old she is. She looks like she could be anywhere between forty-five and fifty-five. She is slim, beautifully dressed, her mass of curly hair is blonde and brown with a little grey in it, her face is lightly made-up and her eyes surrounded by fine lines. She simply looks spectacular.

Later on, I work out that as she was fifteen when her favourite book *Bonjour Tristesse* came out in 1954 she must be at least sixty-five by now. I can't believe it; the woman looks fantastic. She is seductive, elegant, chirpy and above all natural. This is the absolute key to the French way of ageing. In fact women of all ages are expected to look natural. There is nothing more off-putting in France than a woman who looks like she's plastered on make-up and had her hair dyed, whatever her age. (Obviously you can do those things, just don't let the rest of the world know you've done them.)

Sabbia tells me she thinks the most beautiful thing about a woman's face is her experience. 'It's her life,' she says. 'Why should she try to destroy it? A woman of eighty can be chic if she looks after herself, there is no reason why not.' Sabbia shows me pictures of her granddaughter dressing up as we chat. I am still finding it hard to believe this woman is a grandmother. She tells me her greatest beauty secret is that she exfoliates her skin regularly and cleanses her face religiously morning and night. I leave her in her lovely underwear boutique in Saint-Germain and pop to the chemist's for an exfoliating potion before my next meeting. This woman has obviously found the recipe to ageing with grace and I intend to copy it.

The actress Charlotte Rampling will be sixty next year. She has been labelled the thinking man's crumpet and is still incredibly sexy. She lives in France and has adopted a French attitude towards ageing. She has not had plastic surgery and is not considering it. 'Many women are destroying their faces trying to look young,' she says in an interview with the *Sunday Times*. 'Ageing can make you quite beautiful. A few wrinkles here and there but so what?'

Respect, admiration and acceptance of age are nothing new to the French woman. Colette, the writer, was famous for having a string of young lovers who found her irresistible, even in her old age. One of her most popular books, *Chéri*, is all about a young man's love for an older woman. In it, the heroine Léa devotes herself to the amorous education of the beautiful young Chéri. When the time comes for Chéri to marry, he finds it impossible to leave her. Aged forty-nine, she holds more allure for him than his young wife. She is extremely attractive and knows it, as the following quote shows. 'Everyone knows,' Léa would say, 'that a well-made body lasts a long time.'

French men love women of any age. Balzac had many lovers and almost every one was older than him. 'Our young girls are too concerned with making a rich match, passion comes later,' he once said.

According to my friend Henri who is in his early

thirties, his French contemporaries are still going for older women. 'The young ones are so demanding,' he says. 'Especially if they're pretty. They want it all; children, careers, adoring husbands who they wrap around their fingers. A lot of my friends find older women a lot easier to handle and a lot more fun to be with.' So there's hope for us all.

Diane de Poitiers was eighteen years older than her lover King Henri II, but he much preferred her to his wife Catherine de Medici. In fact his wife had trouble conceiving an heir and Diane, realising that an annulment of the marriage and a new queen could compromise her position, used to arouse Henri before sending him to his wife's bed to complete the task. His dynastic duty done he would return to Diane's bed. Catherine eventually became pregnant and bore the king a healthy son. Catherine de Medici couldn't understand her husband's obsession with his ageing mistress and so had a carpenter drill two holes on the floor directly above Diane's bedroom. She and her maid would watch them making love and conceded, weeping, that he 'had never used me so well'.

Diane was one of the first examples of a woman ageing with grace. She always looked after herself; eating mainly fruit, nuts and vegetables. Her regular beauty habits paid off; she was stunning until the day she died.

French women see beauty as something to work on. They start at a young age by protecting their skin from the sun and eating well. 'We see regular and healthy habits as far more effective than layers of concealing make-up,' says my friend Nadine. Even Catherine Deneuve concedes she has to make an effort. 'Today it is hard work,' she said in a recent television interview. 'Up to about thirty it's great, but after that it becomes more difficult, you have to be more careful.'

One thing I started doing is sleeping on my back instead of my side. I wish I had known about this years ago, before a long wrinkle all down the side of my face started developing. Looking back, I can't believe how I did not realise what was causing it. Every French woman I know seems to be genetically programmed not to sleep on her side. After two months of sleeping on my back it seems to be diminishing. At first I found changing my sleeping position impossible. I kept waking up on my side and wondering how I got there. But I have got used to it now. And if I am tempted to sleep on my side I think about the wrinkle from hell which usually inspires me to move pretty quickly.

My Yorkshire friend Jeanette says she is encouraged by the French attitude towards age. 'Back home friends of mine would start to look old as soon as they had children,' she says. 'Here you see people with grandchildren and they still look sexy. They have this ageing thing sussed. They continue to take pride in their appearance, they look polished.'

So it's back to the beauty regime and looking after yourself. If you are going to age gracefully you need to start young. You need to adapt your look with your age so that you always look natural. This will mean lighter hair as you get older and less make-up. You will also have to stay thin. But I don't think you need to be boring.

'You should always follow fashion a bit,' says Inès de la Fressange, who was born in 1957 but looks about twenty five. 'But don't forget your own style. Take some risks, go to some new shops, new places, get ideas from the magazine. But above all don't wander around thinking young people are all terrible and talking about the past all the time. Hang out with young people. Appreciate them. Also appreciate your life with the wisdom that comes with age. If you decide that your life is not so bad and you're actually quite lucky then it becomes a reality. You can go out and hate everybody, hate your age and hate all the things you don't have but it will show; you have the face you deserve.'

There is a lot more pressure now on women to look attractive, no matter their age. In France there is a clothing shop called Comptoir des Cotonniers. It has a very successful advertising campaign where mothers and daughters model their collections. The mothers are just as glamorous as their daughters, sometimes more glamorous. The point they are making is that you can look good even if you're old enough to be someone's mother.

On my next trip to Paris I have a drink with B. We meet in the famous Deux Magots café in Saint-Gemain. I ask him if he finds older women attractive.

'Age has nothing to do with sexiness,' he says. 'Attraction can transcend any age. And nowadays a woman of fifty today is not viewed the same way she was twenty years ago. Forty is no longer middle-aged. Anyone between eighteen and eighty one can wear a well-cut pair of jeans, a T-shirt and jacket and look great. There is no mystery to ageing with grace; it is common sense.'

I don't think plastic surgery is the answer. At least not for me. After the experience of the London party full of freaky-looking women I have cancelled my appointment with Anne Robinson's miracle doctor; I'm going to try ageing the French way. There is something more honest about growing old gracefully. I also think all this stuff is risky. A friend of mine had botox and then had to have eyelid surgery because her eyelids drooped as a result of the botox. This is not a vicious circle I want to get involved in. And for all the pop star Toyah Wilcox's assertions that she is happy with her facelift, I have to say I think she looks most unusual.

The French women I spoke to seem to be sanguine about old age. They don't even seem to dread it. 'I am sure I will be the first grandmother to walk on the moon,' says 'It' girl Hermine de Clermont-Tonnerre. 'But I will have to stay hyper rock and roll.' I am sure she will, without botox.

5

Indispensable Allies

'The most beautiful make-up on a woman is passion.
But cosmetics are easier to buy.'
Yves Saint Laurent

I wonder briefly whether I have finally gone mad. I am
lying in a darkened room, covered in small plastic pots.
These are attached to a machine via big black tubes.
Every two or three seconds a pot sucks in bits of my flesh
and then spits it out. I feel like a dairy cow at milking time.
This torture, or beauty treatment as the French call it, is
meant to reduce cellulite. It is one of several million tricks
French women use to stay thin, young and cellulite free.

For French women, the battle against the bulge doesn't
start in the kitchen; it starts in the perfumery and the

pharmacy. In the perfumery, where I am regularly milked in both senses of the word, you will find exquisite beauty products and perfume. This is where you can buy your Clarins body sculpting cream as well as the latest Lâncome products and Chanel scent. The chemist, pharmacy (or *para-pharmacie*) as the French sometimes call them, is where you will find a different range of products, all essentially with the same aim of keeping you thin and beautiful, but for less money and with perhaps more of a medical than beautifying flavour. 'The packaging is not as nice as the ones you get at the perfumery,' says my friend Aurélie, who works for Chanel. 'But the products are good.'

You only have to walk into a French chemist's to understand a lot about French women's philosophy towards beauty and staying in shape. They are filled with potions and lotions, all designed to make you sleeker, thinner and your skin smoother. As the actress Florence Pernel admits: 'I hate diets, I can't even think about them. I prefer to try creams.'

The French have a great belief in beauty products and would as soon give them up as stop eating baguettes. 'Products that are related to beauty, such as cosmetics and perfume are presented to us as indispensable allies in any conquest, and to refrain from buying them is the equivalent of retiring to a convent,' says French style guru Geneviève Antoine Dariaux, who has written a whole book on how to stay elegant.

I have travelled all over France and wherever I go I always check out the chemist. I love walking into a French chemist's. It doesn't matter what sort of a mood you're in, a French chemist can always soothe you. For me it's the equivalent of Tiffany's, where Holly Golightly would go if she were feeling down in *Breakfast at Tiffany's*. The smells, the vast array of products, the promises on the wrapping of a better, thinner, healthier life with no orange-peel-like-skin all cheer you up. There is really nothing medicinal about a French chemist. Of course you can get prescriptions there, but all the medicine is hidden away behind the counter. What you have on display are countless products that will help you in your battle to gain and maintain the perfect body. You only have to leave with a bag full of jars and you feel thinner already.

And it's obviously not only me who feels this way. According to Brigitte Papin, health and beauty editor of *Madame Figaro* magazine, one in three supplements sold in a French chemist's is a slimming aid.

When I first moved here I thought all these ointments and pills were a waste of money. How on earth could they make any difference to one's body? Surely the only thing that can help is a starvation diet? Brigitte tells me my attitude is 'so English'. She says the French have been using slimming and anti-cellulite creams with great results for over twenty years. She likens me to a woman she met recently in Bordeaux who had brown spots all over her hands and who told her she didn't believe in creams. 'I felt like saying, maybe if you did use them you wouldn't have brown spots all over your hands.' I decide I'd better buy some toning creams immediately.

A beautician I met in Montpellier called Héloïse says they do work, but that you have to put them on every morning and every night for at least a month to see any difference at all. She says you should also use a body exfoliating product once a week so the toning cream has a chance to really penetrate. You should also body brush, especially in the summer. This is just a question of brushing your skin rather like you might your hair, always in the direction of the heart, in order to remove dead skin cells.

But the biggest change I have noticed in myself since we moved here has not been in body care but in face care. In England I didn't really wear make up. I was rather like one of those girls my stock-trading friend Tim in Paris is describing when he says that for a lot of English women 'make-up is something other people do'. I also believed, oh so mistakenly, that if one didn't wear make-up, one didn't have to cleanse one's skin. So I would slap on some cold water in the morning before my face cream (I did at least have that) and then some warm water at night.

All that changed when I moved to France. The first thing that happened was that I went to my local perfumery and made friends with the girls who worked there. Once we got chatting, I realised there was a gaping hole where my skin-care regime should have been. 'What cleanser do you use?' asked the lovely Carolyn, looking crisper than a winter's morning in the Alps in her white uniform and perfectly sleek hair. I told her that as I didn't wear make-up I just used water.

She looked horrified, then sympathetic. I could almost hear the words 'poor deluded woman' running through her head. She told me, very patiently, that even if I didn't wear make-up I still had to cleanse my face every morning and every night. Would I prefer a milk-based cleanser or a water-based one? I smiled inanely. This was getting very technical. Carolyn again took me in hand and said that if I wasn't used to cleansing then maybe one I could use with water would be best, especially as I was at least used to water. Then we had to choose a toner, then an eye cream, then a cream for the lips, then a night cream.

You would think that would be enough. But no. Last time I went to see Carolyn to discuss the pros and cons of the new Dior anti-ageing cream Sharon Stone is marketing she asked how I was getting on.

'Fine,' I told her. 'I've even started to wear make-up.'

'And you're using the same cleanser I gave you?'

'Yes,' I beamed proudly. 'Every morning and evening.'

Carolyn looked horrified. Again. 'But you can't. That's just for cleansing if you don't wear make-up. You have to use one that takes off make-up. Do you realise that if you go to bed wearing your make-up you can age six days in one night.'

In this beauty game you have to keep on your toes at all times. As for the Dior products, Carolyn thinks they're great, but not as great as Ms Stone herself whom she was lucky enough to see at an event she was invited to.

'I've never, ever thought about, you know, other women,' she confided. 'But Sharon Stone, well, she could change my mind.'

My bathroom now looks more like Sophie's, the first French woman I ever met who so impressed me with her array of beauty products. It is filled with jars, creams and exfoliating rubs. And of course a cleanser I use at night to take my make-up off, and another one I use in the morning when I'm not wearing any make-up. Every morning and night I religiously cleanse my face before putting on eye cream, lip cream, day cream or night cream. I also eat supplements that are meant to be anti-ageing and even drink herbal tea that's meant to make your stomach flat (oh please, I know, of course it can't work, but it makes you feel a lot holier than a double latte).

I really don't know whether it all does any good or not, but I'd rather not run the risk of ageing prematurely if I can avoid it. Now that I have got into a routine, it doesn't seem to take so long and what better way to spend five minutes a day than on yourself? The only downside is that my daughters are now mad about creams as well. I came home from town once to be told by our baby-sitter Andrea that my oldest daughter Olivia (age five) had been using my vastly expensive eye cream, on her legs. Cue one huge heart attack.

I can now see how French girls naturally fall into the regime. I was kissing Olivia goodnight one evening when she told me I smelt nice. I said it was my night cream. 'You don't need cream at night,' she said.

'Oh yes you do,' said the new fully-converted, brainwashed me. 'You have a cream for the day and a cream for the night.' 'Yes, and when I'm big like you,' replied Olivia. 'I'll have a cream for the day and a cream for the night too.'

Carolyn from my local perfumery says this subconscious teaching is essential. 'A woman who looks after herself, who takes time to take her make-up off and cleanse is teaching the first gift of beauty to her child,' she says. 'The morning and evening cleansing ritual is the most important beauty tip you can pass on to them.'

French girls start learning about beauty very young. On a trip to Paris this summer I was in Monoprix, a department store in Saint-Germain. A thirty-something Parisian was shopping with her two daughters. She was dressed in black and white; tight-fitting trousers and a matching top. She wore Gucci sunglasses and Gucci sandals. Her hair was subtly streaked and natural looking, her make-up perfect. It goes without saying that she had manicured hands and feet. She paid for an assortment of things including a lip-gloss which I thought at the time looked a little too glaringly pink for her. As soon as it was paid for, one of her daughters, who could not have been more than seven years old, took it out of the bag and started applying it. She had obviously been watching her mother. This was not the cack-handed effort of a child unused to putting on lip-gloss. She expertly glossed her lips with a few quick movements and then admired the effect in the nearest mirror. Just like a girl of seventeen would have done.

Carolyn tells me that the average age for a girl to start waxing her legs in France is eleven years old. I am stunned by this news. Aged eleven, I had no concept of hairiness or non-hairiness. 'Eleven is when they start big school,' says Carolyn. 'They want to look good. I once had a client come in with her nine year old. She screamed and hated it. She was a total tomboy and a bit too young I think.' I dread to think how much money we are going to spend with the local perfumery once all three girls start demanding lip-glosses, leg waxes and facials. Maybe this is why child benefit is so generous in France. I really didn't believe her until my childminder Chantel asked for a morning off to take her daughter Laurie to have her legs waxed. She was twelve at the time. 'It's the age when these things start,' said Chantel, looking very proud, as if she was taking her to her first driving lesson.

For the older client things are looking up. Isabelle Pecenicic, head of Cosmetics at Galeries Lafayette, says there is more and more demand for effective products and they are being launched every five minutes. 'We are being attacked by images of young women everywhere,' she tells me as she shows me around the cosmetics floor of the store. 'Society demands that we stay young and a lot of women do not want to resort to surgery. If you have radiant skin, you don't need it. This of course means you have to cleanse every day. And use good creams.' I ask her if anti-wrinkle creams actually work. 'Of course,' she replies (I suppose she would). 'They not only have a physical effect, but a mental effect too.'

On this at least I agree. It might sound obsessive and slightly pathetic covering myself with unguents and fragrant things. But I feel a lot better for it. I would miss my beauty routine now if I didn't do it. When I travel and my husband isn't there to physically carry the enormous amounts of bottles I now have for this and that part of my body and face, I actually feel slightly deprived. Rubbing gel into your breasts every morning might make them fuller and firmer and it might not. But whatever else it smells lovely and makes you feel good.

And at least nowadays a beauty regime is mercifully easy. Diane de Poitiers, mistress to Henri II of France, was terrified of wrinkles and would sleep sitting up on pillows to reduce them, as well as wear a black velvet mask to prevent exposure to the sun. She would also drink a dreadful sounding mixture of asses' milk, water and liquid gold which she believed kept her young looking. However obsessive I have become since moving to France, this is not an option I have considered, yet.

Not surprisingly the French cosmetics industry is huge. French women are the world's biggest consumers of beauty products. They spend an average of $290 per person on them every year. Around Paris and big cities, women spend around ten per cent of their income on beauty products. This figure is split between make-up items twelve per cent, scents and toners, so-called *parfumerie alcoolique* (thirty two per cent), shampoo and hair care (seventeen per cent), beauty and treatment products (twenty eight per cent), and miscellaneous hygiene products (eleven per cent). According to government figures for 2001, there were almost eight hundred cosmetics companies in France compared with only three hundred or so in the UK. France is the second biggest exporter of cosmetics in the world with a fourteen per cent share of the market worth an annual $91 billion.

By far the biggest figure spent is on perfume. And in France the biggest seller is Chanel. One perfumery worker I spoke to in Paris says that as soon as Chanel launches a new scent she has droves of women coming in saying 'give me the latest Chanel'. They don't even want to try it beforehand. Chanel scents were adored from the start. Diana Vreeland, the editor of American *Vogue* wrote: 'Chanel No 5, to me, is still the ideal scent for a woman. She can wear it anywhere, anytime, and everybody—husbands, beaux, taxi drivers—*everybody* loves it. *No one* has gone beyond Chanel No 5.'

But not all French women always smelt exquisite. Napoleon famously demanded that Josephine should not wash for two weeks before they met so he could enjoy her natural aromas. When she did use scent, Josephine wore a violet-scented perfume (and Napoleon planted violets on her grave, when she died in 1814).

According to an English friend of mine who has lived in the South of France for over twenty five years, most French women didn't use anything to hide their body odour when she first lived here. 'There was a time when you wouldn't pick up a female French hitchhiker. The smell was unbearable,' she says. 'They would have hairy armpits and no deodorant. In fact I don't blame them for that; when we first moved down here, I had to get my deodorant sent from England.' Napoleon would have intercepted the parcel.

But all this has changed. When I first started writing this book, a lot of my English friends said I had to find out whether French women shave their armpits or not. Most of them thought they didn't and were both titillated and scandalised by the thought that all these elegant creatures were wandering around with great bird's-nests under their arms. I can confirm that most French women I know wax under their arms, but that I have seen the odd bird's-nest on the beach. I find it totally disgusting but they don't seem to. I guess it's one of those cultural differences.

Isabelle Pecenicic says that although French women may be true to a brand like Chanel, they are not very true to the individual perfumes. 'They are always being tempted,' she says. 'And very often they will have at least one smell for the summer and another for the winter.' The one exception to this is the actress Florence Pernel who was given a bottle of Lanvin's Arpège by her first boyfriend when she was eighteen. 'It is really an old woman's perfume, but I love it,' she says. 'I will stay faithful to it.'

B, who I meet for a drink on my next trip to Paris, says he finds my scent 'intoxicating'. This is the sort of flattering rubbish French men come out with all the time, but they do appreciate a woman's smell more than the English men I know. 'What a woman should try to achieve with a perfume,' says B leaning closer to me, 'is a hint. A suggestion of seduction and beauty. A lot of women make the mistake of wearing far too much of it and it becomes a turn-off.' For some reason a Coco Chanel quote pops into my head. She was once asked by a young woman where one should use perfume. 'Wherever one wants to be kissed,' Chanel responded. I decide it's time to get the train home.

The other thing I have found myself getting more into since moving here is beauty treatments. Apart from the anti-cellulite one, I also have regular manicures. This was something I used to see as a total waste of money when I lived in England. But now I'm hooked.

There is a saying here: 'She is French to the tips of her nails.' And if you are French, those nails had better be perfect. And we're not just talking fingernails. Your feet have to be properly looked after as well. In Colette's novel *Gigi* the young heroine regularly has her feet checked by her grandmother for any signs of corns. I know it sounds like a terribly sad admission, but I almost always put on foot cream before going to sleep. The first time my husband caught me lying in bed with my legs up in the air rubbing cream into my feet, he thought I'd finally lost it. But you try walking to the bed from the bathroom with your feet covered in thick peppermint moisturising cream: not easy. And of course I go for pedicures, or at least do my toe-nails at home as all this beauty stuff can get expensive.

Most French women who have treatments have them at the beauty parlour or *institut* as they call it here. Sabbia Rosa, the underwear designer, says she goes at least twice a month for waxing or facials or massages. 'I love to have soft skin, so I go for massages with oils. At home I exfoliate all over every other day and moisturise my skin every day. I also get my nails done every week,' she says. Her top beauty tip though is cleanliness. 'Cleanse well every day, I think cleanliness is crucial and the most fundamental thing.'

Not surprisingly, Inès de la Fressange doesn't go in for beauty treatments. 'I'd rather sleep, I'm sure it's better for you,' she tells me. But she agrees with Sabbia on the cleanliness theory. 'I am often surprised to see how badly people take care of themselves. It's not a question of money, everyone can afford a bottle of shampoo,' she says. 'I am sometimes tempted to go up to women and ask why they don't make an effort. If you invite people for dinner, you tidy your house up. Why not make the same effort for yourself?'

The first time I have a facial here I am amazed that Carolyn re-does my make-up once she has finished squeezing my blackheads and covering me in creamy masks. I only ever went for one facial in England but was told not to wear make-up for at least twelve hours after it.

I ask her if it's OK to put make-up on so soon after the treatment. 'Well you can't go out without any on, can you?' is her response. Before I leave her dimly lit treatment room she tells me I should have a facial once a month but exfoliate my skin and have a face pack at home once a week. This is news to me. So far I have lived perfectly happily falling asleep with a face pack on once every five years, but I will do as I'm told and try it.

Edith Cresson, France's former Prime Minister who gained notoriety in England for saying that one in four Englishmen is gay, swears by thalasso-therapy as a beauty treatment. She goes once a year to a spa in Brittany where she stays for two weeks and goes on a strict diet while enjoying all the benefits of the sea and the treatments. 'You come out totally revived,' she says. 'It is extremely good for everything and a very pleasant way to stay in shape.'

Even one of France's most famous feminists, Anne Hidalgo, agrees that looks matter. Anne is the second-in-command at the Paris mayor's office and well known for being a fierce supporter of women's rights. She has the biggest office I have ever seen, with views over the whole of Paris. She herself is tiny, extremely compact and very pretty, giving you the impression she is frail, which she is anything but. 'One is always judged by the style of the envelope, so yes, looks are important,' she says looking very trendy in a hippy-chic outfit. 'But I still guard my right to be as I want to be. If I want to be feminine I am, it's my right and I impose my liberty there as well.'

At the end of the book *Dangerous Liaisons* by Choderlos de Laclos the evil, plotting Madame de Merteuil (played by Glenn Close in the film, in case you haven't read the book) gets smallpox and is disfigured. This is the ultimate revenge of society on a French woman. Excommunication and poverty she would probably have survived, but ugliness is something she cannot overcome. As Madame de Volanges says in one of the final letters: 'Madame de Merteuil was seized with a strong fever, which was at first thought to be the result of the violent situation in which she has been placed; but since yesterday evening it is known that a confluent smallpox of a very bad kind has shown itself. Really, I think it would be fortunate for her if she died of it.'

The message is clear: better dead than ugly. And don't French women know it. Every single one I spoke to told me that looking good is of paramount importance to them. Several, including Inès, even said it is a mark of respect to those around you. In Françoise Sagan's book *Bonjour*

Tristesse, Cécile, the young heroine, sums up the French attitude extremely well. 'I felt vaguely uncomfortable with anyone devoid of physical charms. Their resignation to the fact that they were unattractive seemed to me somehow indecent.'

Doesn't it all get a bit tiring? I mean aren't there days when they want to go out with chipped nail varnish and greasy hair? Do they ever let themselves go? An English friend of mine lives in a chic apartment block near the Eiffel Tower. She says one of her neighbours, a woman of about thirty, won't even take the rubbish out without putting her lip gloss on. In *Bonjour Tristesse* Cécile sees that Anne Larsen, a friend of her father's, has come downstairs on the first day of her holiday perfectly turned out. 'I noticed that she was lightly, but perfectly, made up; apparently she never allowed herself a real holiday.' This seems to be the French attitude. I did try doing the same, but as there is no house within a three-mile radius of ours, putting lip gloss on when taking the rubbish out seemed a bit pointless. But I have to admit that I won't collect the girls from school without first spraying on a bit of scent and glossing my lips. Sad I know, but it's become a habit I can't break.

Sophie Sarkozy, sister-in-law to Nicolas Sarkozy, widely tipped to succeed as the next President of France, maintains they actually enjoy this way of life. 'I don't feel under pressure to look impeccable,' she says. 'I like it. I know English women find it boring but I really do like to look at myself in a mirror and feel good. To me, being well turned out is fundamental and psychologically necessary.' Agnès Cromback, CEO of Tiffany's in Paris agrees. 'If I don't look good, I'm in a bad mood,' she says.

An English friend of mine called Anne who lives in the Auvergne tells me that when she was working in Paris as a teacher she would get the lift up to her classroom on the fifth floor every morning. 'You could always tell which other women in the lift were French and which were English,' she says. 'The French women would be looking straight in the mirror, checking themselves out, and the English would be looking anywhere to avoid it.'

So what other tricks do they get up to in order to make sure they can look in a mirror without wincing? The gorgeous actress Florence Pernel introduced me to the concept of 'peeling' when I went to interview her. Her skin is lovely, almost translucent. She tells me she goes to a dermatologist once every three months and has the top layer of her skin removed. She suggested I call her dermatologist and go for the same treatment. I was tempted but decided to start with a home 'peeling' kit instead, now available from several companies. I found the results pretty good, although sadly I still look nothing like Florence Pernel.

Like all things related to French beauty, hair care also starts in the pharmacy where you can buy little vitamin pills that supposedly make your hair look like Catherine Zeta-Jones's. I don't think they make any difference but then how would you really tell? (The one thing that I have found makes a big difference is the shampoo and conditioner you use.)

The French are very much into what they call '*le brushing*' which means blow-drying. They will go the hairdresser's once a week and get their hair done, not for any particular event but just to make it look good. Sophie Sarkozy even goes to a special hair institute twice a month for an intensive treatment. Marie Sauvage, a colleague of hers who also works in PR, says the hairdresser is her little luxury. 'If my hair doesn't work, it can send me semi-hysterical,' she says. 'Going to the hairdresser always puts me in a good mood.'

This is also something they learn from a very young age. When the girls get their hair cut here (they're aged five and six) they are treated with no less respect and care than I am. They sit down, are given a book to choose a style from, their hair is washed, conditioned, blow-dried and so forth. Bea, who has totally straight hair just like me, will normally ask for something resembling Nicole Kidman on a frizzy hair day. But luckily the hairdresser always manages to convince her that it wouldn't suit her.

French women take their headwear extremely seriously. One of the first women I interviewed for this book was Geneviève de Fontenay who has been running the Miss France competition for the last fifty years. She is a legend in France and famous for not going anywhere without wearing an extremely chic hat. She is known as '*la dame au chapeau*'.

When we meet in a hotel bar in Paris, she tells me she has been wearing a hat since the age of three and that she likes the silhouette it gives her. 'A hat completes a look,' she says, sipping a coffee.

When I walked into the hotel earlier, I suddenly realised I had no idea what she looked like and wondered briefly how I would know who she was. I needn't have worried. Geneviève is your classic vision of a Parisian: sitting extremely straight, immaculately dressed in cream and black, jewellery, red lipstick and (of course) hat. She tells me she does use creams and make-up but doesn't spend hours getting ready. 'Some women take an age,' she says. 'You can't believe how long they spend with brushes and pots.'

One of the topics we discuss is who might be the next President of France. There's been a lot of talk about Ségolène Royal taking the top job I suggest. Geneviève agrees she is a serious candidate but she has two major drawbacks. 'One, she is for the European constitution. Two, she is '*pas bien coiffée*'. Her hair is not well done.

Before you laugh and say what on earth has one's hair got to do with becoming President, you have to remember that for the French presentation is vital. How you look is essential, sometimes more important than what you say or do. They said of Mitterand before he took the top job that he was too short to become President.

If someone is badly dressed or looks shabby, the French will not take them seriously. Letting yourself go physically is seen as a sign that you cannot hold things together intellectually. 'The notion of a French woman being *mal coiffée* is impossible because it shows a lack of attention,' says Michael Worton, Professor of French Literature at University College, London. 'The big thing is the *souci de soi* or care for oneself, in every way. This means brains and looks, you can't let yourself go and be intellectually rigorous.' In other words, the French would sooner forgive an extra-marital affair than a bad haircut. I think briefly about B. Should I have my hair styled before I next see him?

6

La Reine du Beige

*'A dress makes no sense unless it inspires
men to take it off you.'*
Françoise Sagan

I get on the 7.49 at Béziers again and wonder if B will get on at Montpellier. Sadly he doesn't so I catch up on sleep most of the way, and once in town head straight again for Galeries Lafayette. By now I don't even need to tell the taxi drivers at Gare du Lyon I want to go there; they just nod when they see me and head off towards the Boulevard Haussmann. The store is about to open the largest female fashion space in the world, fourteen thousand square metres spread over three floors with two hundred and sixty labels to choose from. What's not to like?

All You Need to Be Impossibly French

I am invited to the launch, which involves shopping with male supermodels (it's such a tough job). Added to which I have an appointment with the store's in-house personal shopper who is going to turn me into a French fashion icon. At least that's the plan.

But the supermodel comes first. Very sweetly the PR girl has arranged for me to meet the most famous of French supermodels, Satya Oblet. You probably don't know his name but would recognise him. He is Indian born with a white beard and spiky white hair. We meet in the champagne bar on the third floor; he is wearing a trendy suit (probably Kenzo, one of his major clients) and looks very suave. He tells me how he got his famous look. 'I was sitting in a bar shortly after I had started modelling,' he says. 'I saw an elderly Indian gentleman walk past with white hair and a white beard. He looked so distinguished. I took out one of my modelling cards and painted my beard and hair with Tipex. I took the card to my hairdresser and told him that was what I wanted to look like.'

Satya and I decide that for him to take me shopping would be ridiculous, as he knows nothing about me. Instead we stay in the bar and chat about French fashion. He thinks it is still dominant, but that the Italians are catching up. He also feels that the French take fashion more seriously than the Brits. 'In France fashion is part of every day life,' says the former Air France purser. 'In England and the US you just dress up when you go out.'

Is he being rude about my appearance?

Maybe it's time to visit Isabelle, the personal shopper. I make my excuses and leave Satya. Walking through the bar I note that the other female shoppers who are taking advantage of the store's 'shop with a male supermodel' offer have taken my lead and are busy plying their shopping partners with champagne. Men never were any good at shopping, but as an idea to get girls to show up and spend money on champagne they are a hit.

Isabelle is not only good at shopping, she does it for a living. She has been the personal shopper at Galeries Lafayette for fifteen years, two years after they began the service. Her job is to help women choose a wardrobe. She greets me with the words 'I had no idea you'd be so tall and beautiful'. Funnily enough I instantly like her.

She takes me into a small room at the back of the second floor and offers me something to drink. She then asks what sort of clothes I'm after. I of course have no idea; I was rather hoping she might tell me. So we chat a little bit about my life, where I work, what I do during a typical day and she then suggests I might like to see some jeans, a jacket, a few tops, maybe a skirt or two.

Once she has an idea of what you want, she goes off to find it and you come back another day. Never one to miss a shopping trip, I decide to go with her instead. 'As a personal shopper I am not interested in labels,' she says as we wander through the fashion floors. 'I am only interested in what looks good on you.' We stop at the jeans bar where you can find just about every style imaginable, although most of them now are low-cut. 'A difficult look for lots of women,' says Isabelle. 'And some of them need to learn to avoid mistakes like trying to look too young. Even in France there is a lot of pressure to look young nowadays, but you just have to accept the way you are and realise that you can still be as attractive, but more feminine and sexy.' Is she trying to tell me something? I hastily replace the pink lace-up jeans with sequins I have been gazing at.

Isabelle suggests four pairs of more sober jeans which we take away with us before moving on to other designers. I ask her to name the most common fashion mistakes clients make. 'People ask for a size thirty eight when they're really a forty two and end up looking ridiculous in a short skirt that is far too tight and heels that make them walk like a duck. And again trying to look too young; fashion nowadays is trendy but it's a mistake to try to look like your daughter or younger sister—dressed in the same clothes, you just won't look your best. The other thing women tend to do is to wear too much make-up, which is not good on older skin.' And I thought French women were perfect.

We choose some little tops (with fairly big prices), a gypsy style skirt and a pink jacket before heading back to Isabelle's office where there is nothing but a full-length mirror, some chairs and hanging space. There, under her watchful eye, I try all the items on. Some of the jeans are terrible, but I love the tops. The skirt is a no and the jacket divine. Isabelle and I agree on everything, now and again she pops out to pick up more goodies. I feel a bit like being a real-life Barbie doll, with an enthusiastic owner dressing you up—brilliant fun.

I ask her what she suggests someone with a limited budget should do when re-vamping their wardrobe. 'Look at your wardrobe before going out,' she suggests. 'There is no point in buying stuff you already have or which is not going to match. Go through your clothes and see what is missing from the basics. Do you have jeans, a skirt, a nice top to go with the jeans, a fitted jacket, shoes with heels and shoes without, a trench-coat? When you go shopping try to mix and match with what you already have.' Isabelle is very keen on accessories and says that a lot of French women's elegance lies in their attention to detail. 'You should always buy the most expensive bag or shoes you can, as they will finish an outfit. Even if you can't afford a Chanel jacket, you can afford to accessorise. I have had my Prada bag for four years now and I wear it with everything, it was a good investment,' she says.

Jewellery is an essential accessory but it doesn't have to be expensive. It was Coco Chanel who first introduced chic Parisians to costume jewellery, sometimes mixing it with the real stuff. Department stores like Monoprix are great for picking up fun and cheap bits to go with whatever outfit you happen to have on. Last time I was in Paris I bought three necklaces and earrings to go with three different outfits for a total of $45.

Isabelle's best advice for successful dressing? 'Colour. If you don't know what colours suit you, then go to a consultant, it's worth it,' she says. I don't know how personal shoppers work in England, but Isabelle's service is free. I suppose they factor in that you will spend more than you would have done without her. At least in my case they were right.

I have arranged to meet B for lunch at a restaurant called Les Fumoirs opposite the Louvre. It is a stylish place, with wooden floors and an almost colonial feel to it. He is already there, looking very French and distinguished.

'I hope you didn't mind me phoning you,' he says. 'I wanted to see how you were getting on.'

I tell him I don't mind at all and explain that my next topic is French fashion.

'You have to remember that fashion is deeply embedded in our culture,' says B. 'It is as important to French women as love.' He explains that his mother was mad about clothes and he grew up traipsing around the streets of Paris with her checking out the latest designs. 'I knew the rue Cambon almost as well as my school.'

The rue Cambon is where Gabrielle ('Coco' is her nickname) Chanel's boutique was first opened in 1921. Chanel hated clothes that hampered movement. 'Some women want to be gripped inside their clothes,' she said. 'Never! When you step inside my dress, you are free.' She established a reputation for relaxed fashions which women could move in, a contrast to the restrained corsets of previous generations. The look was flattering, easy to wear and timeless. They followed the shape of the female body, something only men's clothes had done until she came along.

In 1921 she launched her perfume Chanel No. 5 which became an immediate hit. This was followed by her cosmetics range in 1924. In 1925 she produced her first cardigan jacket which was to become her trademark, closely followed by the little black dress in 1926. This was her heyday; she was the Duke of Westminster's lover and Cecil B de Mille coaxed her to Hollywood where she designed film and stage costumes.

'People often think of Chanel as the classic Parisian woman, chic and stylish, but she was in fact revolutionary,' B tells me. She not only created clothes that women could move and live in, she also created the first boutique where they could buy shoes, bags and cosmetics in one place. Chanel was also the first couture house to offer accessories as well. The *prêt-a-porter* came much later, in 1978.

When World War II started, she closed the shop but moved into the Ritz with a high-ranking Nazi whom she would stay with until his death. In 1944 she was arrested for collaboration with the Germans. She avoided being tarred, feathered and having her hair shorn like others who fraternised with the Nazis and fled to Switzerland. The theory is that the Duke of Westminster asked Churchill to arrange for her release. 'No one knows for sure,' B says.

She remained in self-imposed exile in Switzerland until 1947, when Christian Dior's lavish collection was unleashed on an audience weary of rationing and drabness. He called his clothes *femme-femme* (womanly woman). They were the opposite to Coco Chanel's; heavily structured and boned, lined, padded and impossible to sit down in. It was back to corsets and wasp-waists. 'I adore you,' Chanel is said to have told Dior. 'But you dress women like armchairs.' That might have been so, but women all over the world lapped it up. They loved his flamboyant and feminine style which was in such contrast to the dark, rationed war years.

A further irritation to Chanel was that his two scents, Miss Dior and Diorissimo, had begun to eat away at Chanel No. 5's market share. Finally, in 1954, Chanel decided to make a come-back. It was not a success. The press slated it as retrograde and provincial. But it didn't take long before women again went for her easy and elegant style.

Coco Chanel worked every day until she died in 1971. Every morning she would walk to work from her room at the Ritz. When she left the porter would phone to tell her staff she was on her way. They would then spray Chanel No 5 around the staircase she walked up to get to her studio.

After a lovely lunch B walks me to the Chanel shop in the rue Cambon where I have a meeting with the head of communications, Marie-Louise de Clermont-Tonnerre. She is obviously some relation to my friend the 'It' girl, Hermine. Outside the famous white façade he kisses me on both cheeks, Paris-style, and says he hopes I have as much fun inside as his mother used to.

A doorman lets me into the elegant eighteenth-century building. He is impeccably polite, apologising in advance for any mispronunciation of my name. I hear him say the words '*salon haute couture*'. I don't know why but this makes my heart beat faster. Maybe most women would be excited at the prospect of visiting the Chanel inner sanctuary. The doorman leads me up a staircase which for some reason makes me feel like royalty. It has the most elegant sweep to it and the carpet is plush and thick. There are cut mirrors all along the wall. When you look into them, you can see yourself repeated to infinity. It's not a good place to be when you're having a bad hair day.

I learn that Chanel knocked out the original staircase and designed this art deco one herself. At the top of the stairs the *haute couture* salon opens up in front of me. It is incredibly stylish. Marie-Louise tells me that Karl Lagerfeld redesigned it a year ago. He did a good job; to me it looks like Coco has chosen everything down to the cushions. 'He took as his inspiration the box for Chanel No 5,' Marie-Louise tells me. 'A white box trimmed with black.' Very elegant; in contrast to some of the accessories and clothes on sale in the elegant store below—some of them have a real garish air about them.

There are two colours, cream and black. In fact the cream is a little ambiguous, it could almost be grey. Earlier I asked the doorman who was keeping a watchful eye on me what colour he thought it is. He pondered a moment before replying: '*Blanc cassé*'. Only at Chanel would you find a doorman with such a refined knowledge of colour.

When I ask Marie-Louise, she tells me that of course it is cream. Chanel was known as '*la reine du beige*' (The queen of beige). Silly me. The wooden floors are black varnish with cream carpets. There are leather sofas long enough to sleep top to toe with at least three people in, *chaise-longues* and armchairs, all in the same colour scheme. The coffee tables are black wood with smoked black glass on top. Even the books on the tables match the colour scheme. They are about the house of Chanel, in cream and black. I have an inexplicable urge to draw all over the room with a red felt-tip pen.

There are two rooms off this main salon. One of them

houses the season's collection, which is safely locked away in glass wardrobes. Marie-Louise explains that in Chanel's day you would never see the clothes on a hanger, they would be shown by models. 'The models would parade the collections every day at half past three,' she says. 'Chanel would sit on the fifth step of the staircase leading up to her apartment and watch them mirrored in the glass.'

I ask Marie-Louise how much it would cost me to come and have a classic Chanel suit fitted. She prevaricates and says it's very expensive. I want to know how much. 'I can't tell you in euros,' she says. 'But around 150,000 francs.' So nearly $28,000. One in every colour, please.

Chanel is practically the last house in Paris to do *haute couture*. Dior, Givenchy, Ungaro, most of the big names have stopped. Marie-Louise tells me they still have around two hundred *haute couture* customers; half from the Americas, north and south, and half from Europe. On the floors above the salon a hundred seamstresses work to put together their orders. 'We are very careful when there is a big occasion like the funeral of Prince Rainier or Prince Charles's wedding that no two clients show up in the same outfit,' says Marie-Louise. 'The big difference nowadays is that it is not the husbands or lovers that pay for the clothes, it is the women themselves.'

Next we go up a floor to Chanel's apartment. She didn't actually live at rue Cambon, she lived at the Ritz, but this is where she received her friends and lovers, among them

Picasso, Stravinsky, the Duke of Westminster and Cecil B de Mille. This is also where she would carry out private fittings for friends like Mme de Rothschild and the actress Jeanne Moreau. Her suite at the Ritz is still there. It is called the Coco Chanel Suite.

The apartment is made up of an ante-room, a sitting room, a dining room and a bathroom. The furniture and décor is plush. The most amazing thing is that the whole place is packed with antique screens, some of which Chanel has actually cut holes in to make way for doors. 'She used them like wallpaper,' says Marie-Louise. 'That's the ultimate luxury.'

We go up a floor to Chanel's studio. Her door is one of the things that Marie-Louise, who has worked there since 1971, the year Chanel died, fought to keep. It is yellowing and shabby compared with the rest of the décor but on it is written MADEMOISELLE in black capital letters and *privé* underneath. She was known as Mademoiselle within her empire and in fact still is. My friend Aurélie who works for Chanel still refers to her as Mademoiselle.

Her studio now belongs to Karl Lagerfeld, who has been the chief designer for Chanel since 1983. He has two vast desks and a very modern black and white portrait of Chanel on the wall. There are some model-looking types hanging around, or maybe they're designers. Whatever else, they're very young and very thin. Best to get out before depression sets in.

The only place Marie-Louise won't let me into is the workshops, she says it will disturb the workers. I wonder irreverently whether the floors above are in fact full of cobwebs (cream of course) and all the clothes are now made in China, before quickly suppressing this sacrilegious thought about the holiest of holies.

We go back to her office which is filled with photographs of the great lady. We talk about *haute couture*. She concedes that it is no longer big business. I ask her why they keep doing it. 'You and I wouldn't be here today if it weren't for the fact that Chanel had done *haute couture*,' she says. 'Why would we abandon it? It would be unfaithful and like erasing our roots.' Interestingly Mademoiselle herself had nothing against abandoning her own roots. She had a major fall-out with Louise de Vilmorin, a writer, when the latter refused to lie about Chanel's humble origins in a biography of her. The book was never written and litigation over the advance ensued.

I ask Marie-Louise if Karl would ever design anything for a single person. 'It's most unusual,' she says. 'He has designed for Nicole Kidman and Caroline of Monaco, but these were exceptions. What you can do is reserve the sole right on a design, you can be the only person in the world to wear say a particular dress, but of course that costs a lot of money.' As does everything associated with *haute couture*. According to Agnès Cromback at Tiffany's *haute couture* is now beyond the means of the French. 'France lets the foreigners dream and enjoy what we have that is extraordinary, but not the French,' she says. 'They simply can't afford it any more.'

Fashion is deeply ingrained in the psyche of the French woman. She has grown up with all these names; they are part of her history and her culture. It is hardly surprising that grunge never took off in France and punk could never have happened here. If you're a French woman you have, just like its fashion and cosmetics industry, a logo to live up to.

People expect French women to look good. Is this why they do?

Inès de la Fressange, a former Lagerfeld muse, agrees there is something in the French make-up that makes them predisposed to fashion, but she does not think that French women are somehow more chic than other women. 'Really I shouldn't say that,' she admits. 'I have been trading on that reputation for twenty five years, and have been very happy to do so. But in reality it's an old cliché.'

Geneviève de Fontenay, the Miss France doyenne, agrees with her. 'There is not the refinement there was in the 50s and 60s,' she says. 'Now the fashion is for ripped jeans, not couture. We have lost something in France. If Monsieur

Dior could see what women look like nowadays, he would turn in his grave.' Sophie Sarkozy insists that French women still have an indefinable flair. 'It is not a cliché. Just go to the Avenue Montaigne and you'll see it there. There is always, no matter what time of day or night, a girl there who epitomizes what we think of as the classic Parisian. She will be thin, perhaps not ultra elegant, but fashionable. And above all she will have an allure. It's genetic and we French have it, rather like the Balinese dancers, it's not something you can learn.'

In fact the French never forget about fashion, even in adversity. *Elle* magazine's coverage of the riots against the law reforming the youth employment law focused on what is saw as the most crucial aspect: what rioters were wearing. 'There is a boom in the rubbish-bin-dress,' it noted. 'The symbol of the throw-away salary.' I must pick one up on my next trip to Paris.

I wander down the famous Avenue Montaigne the next day to see who is right. It is early and raining so I don't actually expect to see anyone, let alone a style icon. Dior is just opening up. Its vast shop spans an entire block and everywhere along the avenue window washers are busy wiping off yesterday's grime. I see a couple of African-looking ladies scurrying off to work, a few men in suits, and then, there she is. Your classic, but perfect, Parisian. She is wearing a cream hat, black trench-coat, cream trousers and high-heeled cream shoes. The only splash of colour is a

Hermès (at least I assume it's Hermès) scarf tied loosely round her neck which is cream, black and pink. She is carrying some medical-looking documents and chatting on the phone. Minutes after her another one appears. This one is more colourful; she wears a pink trench-coat, cream trousers and high heels. She is heavily pregnant but looks totally chic. I spend another half an hour scouring the avenue for classic Parisians. No more appear, but Sophie's point has been proven.

Most French women do not do their shopping on the Avenue Montaigne. They go to small shops where they can find bargains or chains like Zara and Hennes. When I last saw Aurélie, my friend who works for Chanel, she was wearing a lovely white shirt. I assumed the shirt was from the latest Chanel collection. Not at all. 'It's from Naf Naf,' she told me proudly. Unlike Americans who like to show off their labels, French women take a perverse pride in trying to buy good things from cheap shops.

'In the US if you wear the latest Prada jacket, then everyone knows you're wearing the latest Prada and that's important to you,' says Inès de la Fressange. 'Here if you pay a French woman a compliment for an item of clothing, she'll say 'oh it's an old thing', in a way make an excuse for it.' The main reason for this is that it is viewed as vulgar to show off your wealth in France. Also the tax man is less forgiving of success than he is in Anglo-Saxon countries. There is also a social stigma attached to success and you'd be better off carrying a Hermès bag with the label on the inside than on the outside.

The historian and psychoanalyst Elisabeth Roudinesco suggests that one of the reasons success is frowned upon in France is that whereas in Anglo-Saxon countries we identify with the person who has made it and want to be like him or her, in France they identify with the person who has suffered due to their success. 'We hate success,' she says. 'As soon as you're successful here, you're attacked. If you're rich, beautiful and a genius then forget it. As a woman you're better off being an intellectual with Margaret Thatcher's looks than Ava Gardner's.'

After my walk down the Avenue Montaigne I head back to Galeries Lafayette for a meeting with Pascale Camart, head of women's fashion. I ask her about the classic French style we all want to emulate. She tells me the Chanel look is 'a lovely image, but not representative of the French woman any more'. She shows me around the three floors of fashion and a lot of it is very trendy, there is lots of hippy chic.

Pascale herself is wearing a gypsy-style skirt, huge necklace, flouncy shirt and shawl; she looks great. So is it all over for Chanel? 'No, of course not,' she says. 'But nowadays you would wear a Chanel jacket with a pair of jeans and white T-shirt. French women want to be more fashionable, more adventurous. Fashion is more amusing now. It is fun, you mix colours and materials. It is all about how you carry it and accessorise it. But you have to practise it every day if you're going to keep up.'

It all sounds exhausting. I ask her how long she has worked in fashion and what keeps her motivated. 'I have been here for eighteen years,' she says. 'I love the renewal, discovering things, I'm always looking for something new that will surprise and be different.' She tells me she shops for clothes at least once a week. I ask her how many skirts she owns. She is coy about the exact figure but does admit she has a whole room at home dedicated to her clothes. 'I love clothes,' she says. 'I know it's my job and I have to look good, but I truly love them.'

It's time to get the train home. I say goodbye to Pascale, who is relieved as it gives her some time to shop, and I jump in a taxi. On the train a girl in her mid-thirties sits next to me. We start chatting and I can tell from her accent she doesn't spend her spare time on the Avenue Montaigne. She is called Laurine and is from Béziers. She has worked in Paris but has now gone back to take over her family wine business.

Rather like I have changed since I moved to France, she tells me she has changed since she moved from Paris. 'I used to go to the hairdresser once a week, have my nails done, eyebrows plucked etcetera,' she says. 'It all seemed so terribly important. But since I came back down south, I don't bother. I figure a woman is a little like a bottle of wine. Her label is not important; it's what is inside that counts.' I ask her if she thinks fashion is important. 'No, not at all,' she says. 'Fashion is something the Parisians have time to worry about. I am too busy trying to sell my wine.'

I agree with her. Although I feel trendy, attractive, and happy in the clothes Isabelle has chosen for me, I don't think I will ever become as obsessive about fashion as some of the women I have met.

But strangely enough, even though Laurine maintains she does not take an active interest in fashion, she is very stylish in her jeans and black polo top with her hair tied back in a pony-tail. She may not be what a Parisian would call chic, but she certainly wouldn't look out of place in Knightsbridge or New York.

7

Beyond One's Control

'My friends, there are no friends.'
Coco Chanel

'The thing about your girlfriends,' my French friend Sylvie says to me as we are having lunch in a restaurant in Montpellier, 'is that sooner or later they end up sleeping with your husband or boyfriend.' This seems to me an extraordinary statement. 'But I've never even met your husband,' I protest. 'Exactly,' she responds. 'That's why you haven't met him.'

Sylvie's attitude is apparently typical of French women, most of whom are insanely jealous and suspicious. One of the reasons they spend most of their time trying to look so good is to stop their girlfriends seducing their husbands.

There is much more rivalry and much less solidarity between them than between English girlfriends. In England it's a given that you're not going to try to seduce your best friend's boyfriend; here it is assumed that you are.

Nicolas, a French male friend of mine who lives in London, says that the women are right to be anxious. 'French women do have girlfriends, but they usually end up sleeping with their friend's boyfriends. It just happens. Marital infidelity also happens mainly with people you are close to. The French don't want to resist their instincts or passions. It's not in their genetic make-up.' As the Vicomte de Valmont says in the book *Dangerous Liaisons*: 'It is beyond my control.'

Women avoid bringing other single women into their lives, even if they are close friends. Sabbia Rosa tells me that she has a lot of girlfriends, but despite the fact that her husband works abroad most of the week, she is never invited to their homes alone. 'I don't know what they are scared of, it's not as if I'm a great seducer,' she tells me as we sit in her boutique in Saint-Germain. 'But women on their own are definitely seen as a threat.'

Nathalie, a friend of mine who lives in Bordeaux, tells me that when she split up with her long-term boyfriend, she decided to give dinner parties for friends to take her mind off things. 'We had been together for almost ten years,' she says. 'So it took a bit of getting over.' She would invite married couples she knew but she would be on her own. After a few dinners one of her friends phoned her and said: 'I wish you would stop inviting us over the whole time, you're never going to get one of our husbands.' Nathalie was horrified. 'I wasn't inviting them over to seduce their husbands, but that is the mentality here.'

Alexandra, my best friend in France, has as far as I know not yet tried to seduce my husband. She lives about twenty minutes away from us and has two children, one of whom is my daughter Olivia's best friend. Although we are very close, I think there is always something missing when you don't share the same culture, or more importantly language. If you compare English and French girls though, I do think she has been as open and friendly as any English girl would have been. Although she does drink a lot less and is probably a little more formal.

But as yet I have not made any really close friends who are actually from the Languedoc region where I live, and nor has Alexandra. She is from Nantes and is viewed as being as foreign as I am. In fact in the Languedoc you are better off being from England than from Paris—they really loathe Parisians.

Apart from me, Alexandra has two other close friends;
one Dutch woman and one French-Canadian woman who
went to university in Newcastle. As a woman I think it's
tougher to infiltrate French society. My husband has made
lots of friends just by getting on his bike, but there are no
equivalents of the male cycling club for women. French
women just don't really seem to like hanging out together.

'It' girl Hermine de Clermont-Tonnerre says she has
very few friends and that most of them are foreign.
'French women are so jealous,' she says. 'I can't stand it.'
She says that before she got together with her British
husband Alistair, her girlfriends paid him no attention.
'They would barely say hello,' she says. 'Then when we
got together, they looked at him differently. Suddenly he
was more interesting, as soon as he became my boyfriend
they wanted to know all about him, they thought he must
have something special. It was Alistair darling this and
Alistair darling that. Their first aim is to destroy the
couple.'

This might seem insane to an English girl, but Hermine
is not alone in experiencing the destructive power of the
French female. Caroline Wachsmut, a stunningly beautiful
Swiss girl who has her own skin care label called Doux Me,
says she finds the French attitude very hard to live with.
'The women are constantly comparing who has the best
marriage, the best clothes and so on,' she says. 'They invite
you to their homes because they're nosey and want to find

out all about you. And as soon as things are going well in your work life they try to destroy your relationship by circulating rumours that your husband is being unfaithful or whatever. They can't stand success; it's a very Parisian mentality.'

According to my Yorkshire friend Jeanette in Montpellier this attitude is not limited to Paris. 'The thing you have to remember about France,' she says. 'Is that women are still oppressed by men and that women defend themselves and get what they want by seducing men. Not sleeping with them but flirting. The downside to this is that it affects their relationship with other women.'

There is a lot more competition between women here than I ever noticed back home. One extraordinary thing is that if you are with a French girl and you see a good-looking couple walk down the street, she will be looking at the girl.

I wondered at first if this was a deep-rooted lesbianism but am told that is not at all the case. It's all about checking her out, seeing how she's dressed, what bag she's carrying, how well her nails are done and so on. By the time I have worked out how fit the guy is, my French friends have totted up the net worth of the girl's outfit and made a mental note of her nail colour.

I have also found that some of my friends lack the solidarity my English and American girlfriends have. Colette puts it very well in her book *The Cat*. Claudine the heroine is talking to her husband who asks her why she doesn't see her friends more. "'Girls,' she explained with some bitterness, "Girls don't stick together decently. There's no solidarity. It's not like all you men.'"

French women, however, do stick up for their men. On 16 March 1914 Henriette Caillaux, wife of Joseph Caillaux, a French cabinet minister, walked into the office of Gaston Calmette, the editor of *Le Figaro* newspaper. The newspaper had been attacking Caillaux's politics and also publishing letters from him to his first wife when she was his mistress and married to someone else. It had promised to publish more. Mme Caillaux walked into the office, said 'you know why I have come' and then fired a gun six times, killing the editor. This happened on the eve of the World War I, but her trial dominated the front pages. She was eventually acquitted; her crime deemed a *crime passionel*, a crime of passion.

But when it comes to the sisterhood they're not really with it. On the morning of her fifth birthday party Olivia turned to me and asked: 'Which other childrens (sic) are coming?' I had invited Alix, a friend of hers from school, a friend called Emmanuelle and her daughter and of course Bea, Olivia's sister. My friend Alexandra was away. Olivia seemed happy with the guest list so we carried on inflating the Barbie castle. About two hours before the party, Carolyn (Alix's mother) called to say that Alix was ill and couldn't come. I asked if maybe her younger sister would like to come instead. She said no it probably wasn't a good idea.

I immediately called Emmanuelle to make sure she was coming with her daughter. At least there would be one child at the party Olivia wasn't related to. She sounded very lacklustre and said that no, she didn't think they could make it because her baby had been up in the night and she was feeling tired. I explained that there would be no children at all at Olivia's birthday (apart from her own sister) if they didn't come, but this didn't seem to make an impression.

I was totally amazed, this would never have happened in England. But after I got over my initial fury, I realised that this was just her way, she didn't see it as a big deal and would have been amazed that I did.

The party turned out all right. When Carolyn heard that there would be no other children, she dragged Alix from her sickbed and bundled her in the car. The girls had a lovely time bouncing on the Barbie bouncy castle—at the sight of the vision in pink Alix made an instantaneous recovery. I am eternally grateful to Carolyn who obviously has some girlie English gene hidden away somewhere.

Emmanuelle's reaction was basically an honest one: she didn't feel like coming. This off-hand frankness a lot of French women have can make them come across as unfriendly or snotty. I remember when I came back from London with a new haircut a few months ago. My friend Alexandra looked at me and asked if I'd had my hair cut.

'Yes,' I replied.

'I preferred it before,' said my best friend.

At the time I thought it was quite rude, but on reflection it was just being honest. Although it's a kind of honesty we overly-polite Brits are unlikely to employ the way the French would.

But it is the girlie thing that is the key to the difference in friendships here. You don't see girls going out together, drinking wine and talking about their boyfriends. You might see two friends together but I have never seen a cluster of girls hanging out and laughing uproariously like they do in wine bars and pubs all over the UK and US. The dancing around the handbag syndrome seems to have bypassed the French female entirely. 'I just don't understand what you're all on,' says Nathalie who lived in London before moving to Bordeaux. 'There is nothing more boring than hanging out with a lot of girls, what's the point in it?'

Dorothée Werner, a journalist with *Elle* magazine in Paris, thinks the difference goes back to childhood. 'Education is much more mixed here,' she says. 'We were brought up with the idea that we were the same as boys in the sense that we can play football and dress like them. I think this makes us less girlie and fragile. We are more independent from the group.' Her colleague Marie-Pierre Lannelongue agrees. 'I also think sex differences are natural here,' she says. 'We are relaxed about it early on. Children aged four talk about marrying each other; they are into the game very early.'

I compare my step-children who were four and six when we were living in England and the little ones, who are four and five now. I certainly don't remember as much talk about love, kissing and marriage from Hugo and Julia as I now get from Olivia and Bea.

My daughter Bea often comes home from school and announces that, for example, Nicolas and Héloïse have 'kissed on the lips' and that they're 'in love together' and planning to 'marry together'. She is four years old. Olivia, aged five, has already decided not to get married but to live with Daddy for the rest of her life. So far I haven't heard a single 'boys are stupid', which I did hear a lot from Julia (and vice versa from Hugo) but then maybe that was because they were close in age. Our son Leonardo is a couple of years younger than the girls so doesn't annoy them too much, except when he runs off with their Barbie dolls—a rather worrying habit I am hoping he'll grow out of when he meets a real one.

'The point is,' says Dorothée, 'that the foundation of

society in France is that men and women know they are different but feel equal. Therefore the whole relationship is more natural. The men are also less of a caricature than in England where you have the classic bloke in the pub.'

The psychoanalyst and historian Elisabeth Roudinesco agrees. 'I find relationships between men and women here much more civilised,' she says. 'In Canada, for example, it's got to the stage where a male psychoanalyst won't take on a female client for fear of being accused of harassment, it's ludicrous.'

I remember meeting a girl called Marie in Paris who told me that all her friends were men. She was twenty five and said she had always found men easier to get along with.

The more I learn about French women, the more I can see why. I mean why would you want to hang out with people that are secretly praying for you to put on weight, or trying to sleep with your husband? It's much more fun if their husbands are trying to sleep with you.

I phone B to ask him whether he thinks men and women can ever really be friends. Remember that line in *When Harry met Sally*? 'What I'm saying is that men and women can't be friends because the sex part always gets in the way. No man can be friends with a woman he finds attractive. He always wants to have sex with her.' Is this the case in France? B responds that he has had lots of women friends and that he has wanted to have sex with all of them, but that it has in no way affected their relationship. So that's that then.

My husband has made a French female friend down here. He had never had a female friend back home. At least not one that lived in the same country. He has one who lives in Argentina, which I figure is a safe distance.

But his new friend is younger than me, voluptuous, has long dark hair and, most scarily, works in the wine industry. My husband is mad about wine. He goes sailing with her, in fact once even ran aground on a boat with her and came home at three o'clock in the morning. Luckily, our daughter Julia was with him so I don't think anything happened. Also she smokes, which he hates. But I have to say I am mildly irritated by their friendship.

Am I turning French? I decided the best way to try to avoid her seducing him was to befriend her. She and I get along very well, but I don't know if that would stop her. The French have a weird, if rather charming, attitude towards fidelity. Love, or lust, excuses everything. I can quite imagine a French woman having lunch with you one day and sleeping with your husband the next. As Françoise Sagan says in *Bonjour Tristesse* fidelity is 'arbitrary and sterile'.

I wonder whether French women get lonely. This

fierce competition must get tiresome. Don't they ever want to call a truce?

Simon, an English friend of mine who is married to a French woman, says it is a nightmare for them. He met his wife in Paris. They both worked in offices close to the Opera with vast windows. He could see his wife-to-be sitting at her desk from his office. They started waving to each other and eventually he engineered a 'chance' meeting on the street below.

'Being a classic Parisian she told me she was far too busy to see me for two weeks,' he tells me over lunch one day. 'Then we got together and have now been happily married for almost ten years.' He says he finds his wife's attitude towards other women astounding. 'If my wife meets someone who looks good and is thin, then she immediately loathes her,' he says. 'There seems to be constant competition, to see who is the thinnest, the most successful, the most beautiful. There is a rivalry over men and money that you don't get with the Brits, who seem somehow more sisterly.' There was a TV show on here recently called Clara Sheller. In one scene Clara is talking about her husband to two other mothers. Clara's husband is perfect; a cook, man about the house, kind, considerate and so on. The other women instantly hate Clara. They only become friendly again when she tells them he is in fact homosexual and she got pregnant accidentally.

Another English friend of mine who lives in Lyon with

his French wife says French women are not good at making friends.

'I wish more than anything that my wife had someone she could really talk to, confide in and really relax with,' he says. 'She meets people and they hit it off but after a few months something will go wrong. If she meets a nice-looking woman, her guard is immediately up and there is always a post mortem after evenings with friends. I used to say "hang on a minute, aren't these people friends of yours?", now I just let it slide.' When I asked my friend Jeanette in Montpellier how she would define a French woman who was more like an English woman, she replied, 'One who is interested in being friends with women. Or a relief,' she joked, 'because there aren't many of them.'

According to Michael Worton, Professor of French Language and Literature from University College, London, French culture is much more family-oriented than the British one, so there is not such a need for friends. 'In the UK, the family is no longer the dominant factor,' he says, 'whereas in certain parts of France it still is. Thus the close relationships will be between aunts, cousins, sisters and so on.'

That explains why French women don't go in for the girlie thing. They prefer to hang out with their relations. And according to Nicky, an English friend who lives down here and is married to a Frenchman, their friends almost become their relations. 'They make friends at a very young age,' she says. 'And they stick with them throughout life, whether they like them or not.' Perhaps it is due to the fact that they don't move about as much as the British and Americans do.

In some ways I have become more French. A friend of mine is coming over soon and we're going to spend a weekend at a country club close to here. She was talking to my husband the other day and he said it sounded like we were going to have a nice weekend. 'Yes, it'll be great' she replied. 'We'll get pissed.' She sounded jolly excited about the prospect, but for me the thought of sitting about drinking all evening is no longer as appealing as it once was. The British drinking culture now amazes me. I went to a dinner party the other night and there was one drunk person. And guess what? She comes from Surrey. 'At every wedding I've ever been to, the first person to end up drunk, fully-clothed in the swimming pool is always the English guy,' says Hermine de Clermont-Tonnerre.

The upside to this is that the Brits and Americans are great fun to hang out with, something a lot of the French are not. They don't seem to have that 'laugh at yourself' gene we have and which makes us so endearing. If I had to choose whether to spend an evening with a group of French women or a group of English women, I would always go for the latter, even though I might run the risk of a hangover.

8

Bonjour paresse

'There is no time for cut-and-dried monotony.
There is time for work. And time for love.
That leaves no other time.'
Coco Chanel

No French woman willingly works. This is why the country is full of grumpy sales assistants and waitresses. French women have better things to do with their time, like waxing their legs and seducing other people's husbands. As a male friend of mine who is married to a French woman says: 'They don't see it as an obligation, it is their choice. Theirs is a 'if I want to work I will, if I don't then I won't' kind of attitude. They expect the man to work.'

Of course the French working week is not really geared towards work. If you live in rural France, for example, every Monday is a bank holiday. The banks are closed (of course) as are most shops. When we first moved here I wondered if we were commemorating General de Gaulle's death, birth or overall brilliance as I wandered around town on a Monday trying to fill my empty shopping basket. This Monday closing is rather nice once you get used to it, it eases you into the week gently. Then of course you have Wednesday when there is no school so that practically becomes a holiday too. As there's not much point in getting stuck in work on a Tuesday just for one day, that only really leaves Thursday and Friday morning. So rather a peaceful working week, into which it is hard to cram the required thirty-five hours. The calendar doesn't help either. You start in January which of course coincides with skiing season, so that's a write-off. Then you do a bit of work followed by Lent and Easter. You can then get a couple of weeks in before the first of May, which of course being the workers' day, you do no work on. Once June arrives everyone is gearing up for *Les Grandes vacances*. These happen in July and August, so even if you want to work you can't, as there is no one else around. Then of course you have the *rentrée* in September when everyone goes back to school and work. That takes a few weeks to settle in from by which time you have to prepare for Christmas.

Until I moved here the idea of not working had never

occurred to me. In Britain and the US that is all anyone does. You are defined by what you do. Sometimes I ran across women who did not work, who did not look after their children, in fact who did nothing at all. But they were seen as people to avoid, vaguely suspect in their obvious lack of work ethic or ambition. Now I have a good friend who has about as much work ethic as Max, my cat.

Emmanuelle of course has a lot more to worry about than Max. She has two small children to look after. But what amazes me about her though is her attitude. She talked to me a couple of years ago about becoming a journalist. This was in June. I encouraged her. 'It's a great idea,' I told her. 'Why not go on a course or try to get an apprenticeship with someone?'

'Oh no, it's too late now,' she told me. 'It's not worth doing anything until the *rentrée*.' The *rentrée* happens in September and it's the start of work and school after the summer holidays. I have now seen two *rentrées* come and go, and Emmanuelle is still doing nothing about getting out of the house and into a job. She is one woman who would have welcomed the Vichy government law of 11 October 1940 which excluded married women from working in certain sectors.

Some French people share Emmanuelle's lack of work ethic even when fully employed. *Bonjour Paresse* (Hello Laziness), the publishing sensation of 2004, is a user's guide for the idle worker. It was written by Corinne Maier, an economist who works part-time (naturally) at Electricité de France. Maier advocates getting your revenge on the company that employs you by doing as little as possible. She tells *Le Monde* in an interview how the book 'will explain why it's in your interest to work as little as possible'.

When the book was published it looked likely to sink without a trace until a front page article in *Le Monde* revealed that EDF is planning disciplinary action against Maier for 'failing to respect her obligations of loyalty towards the company'. After that it became a bestseller, with hundreds of French workers lapping up her ten commandments for bored and lazy workers.

Her first commandment is: 'You are a modern-day slave. There is no scope for personal fulfilment. You work for your wages at the end of the month, full stop.' Number three is as follows: 'What you do is pointless. You can be replaced from one day to the next by the cretin sitting next to you. So work as little as possible and spend time (not much, if you can help it) cultivating your personal network so that you're untouchable when the next restructuring comes around.'

I contacted Ms Maier's publishers about an interview but they never got back to me. Maybe they have taken her advice to heart and were too busy doing nothing.

Corinne Maier works for France's public sector, which employs one in four of all workers. I read in an article recently that when asked what they would most like to do when they leave university, seventy five per cent of students say they want to become civil servants. How many students in the UK dream of becoming civil servants? The problem with France is people are not encouraged to become entrepreneurs. They don't seem to have the same attitude towards work the Brits and Americans have. The idea of a safe job for life where you actually work less than thirty five hours a week (civil servants work on average twenty eight hours a week) is great. You do your job badly and live life to the full. You can't be fired and there is no need to use your brain.

I often get the impression people are working here because they have to, not because they want to. As the 'It' girl Hermine de Clermont-Tonnerre says: 'If you go to a restaurant and ask politely for some sugar, the waitress will come and slam it down in front of you. It's outrageous; they have no idea how to offer a service.'

French education is incredibly structured. Some say this is to blame. An essay will not ask for your personal opinion, rather demand the pros and cons of the argument which other people have come up with already. This makes people less imaginative and less independent from a very early age. Liz Rosilio, a documentary maker who was educated at the Lycée in South Kensington and at university in Paris, says she was one of the only students to live away from home. 'Even though we were all around twenty-one,

I was the only one to have my own studio,' she says. 'The others all lived with their parents, ate with their parents and had practically never been to a supermarket.'

Corinne Maier claims that French people are really not interested in their jobs. 'It is *de rigueur* to claim that you work because your job interests you,' she tells *Le Monde*. This work-ethic is not confined to the public sector. An English friend of mine who works for a law firm in Paris. 'You can always tell the French girls from us Brits,' she says. 'At ten to six they start packing up their pencils and at six o' clock on the dot they're out of there. It's only the Brits that are full of beans and willingness.'

The French work less than most other nationalities. In 2004 the OECD reported that the French work twenty four per cent fewer hours now than they did in 1970. Ms Maier for example 'works' only two and a half days a week, which is not uncommon. Women are also given huge amounts of time off (normally around four to six months paid but they can claim up to three years unpaid) if they have babies. The company they work for has to keep their job open for them to come back should they choose to.

Legislation has made employing women distinctly less attractive. 'I think we have protected women to such an extent that it works against them,' says Agnès Cromback, CEO of Tiffany's in Paris. 'If you want a career, you can't just say stop to your boss and expect the company to stagnate. Recently an employee at another company had twins and now she is back after six months demanding Wednesdays and Fridays off.' The statistics perhaps reflect this. In France only three per cent of companies are headed by women. In the UK the figure is closer to eleven per cent.

In the political arena at least, French women are quite high profile. They even had a female prime minister, Edith Cresson. I go up to Paris to meet her and various other political high flyers.

Imagine a female English MP. She is short, broad and badly dressed. Her hair looks like a dead badger that has been dumped on her head. She wears little or no make-up. Let's not even think about her shoes and handbag. She is called Clare Short or Ann Widdecombe. She is serious and she is plain.

This is what I am expecting the sunny morning I go to meet Ségolène Royal. Mme Royal is a member of the French *Assemblée Nationale* and President of the Poitou-Charentes Region. This is no ordinary MP. She is often mooted as a possible future President of France (with the father of her four children taking on the lesser role of prime minister). She proved she is able to do battle with powerful politicians when she took the Poitou-Charentes seat from former prime minister Jean-Pierre Raffarin.

I sit at the table in her room, waiting for her to finish a conversation I am listening to on speaker-phone. She is giving some (male) minion a hard time about drumming up support for the pro-Europe vote and spending funds on non-essential items during this essential election campaign. This is just a few weeks away from the referendum on the European constitution. I look across the table to where she will be sitting. There are two items waiting for her. Some elegant note paper with her name printed on it and a lip gloss. Even the most serious career women in France don't forget that looking good is important.

Eventually Ségolène wafts in, immaculately dressed in a grey suit with a cream silk shirt and scarf. She looks incredible. Slim, elegant and perfectly turned-out; your typical French dream woman. How does she do it?

'I don't,' she tells me. 'It is an ongoing process. Now that the children are a bit bigger, they look after each other. I think that is one of the advantages of having so many. But it is true that I have work and no hobbies, just the family. It's a choice and a passion.' Ségolène looks like the editor of a fashion magazine or successful television producer. I ask her how important appearance is to her.

'I represent a region,' she says. 'I can't just put on jeans and running shoes. I have to be well presented at all times.' In her view, elegance has as much to do with culture as what you wear. 'I think French culture gives us a sense of elegance, there is a harmony which inspires us.' And the top beauty tip from one of France's most high-profile politicians? 'Sleep,' she says. 'You have to sleep to be beautiful. And stay positive.' She and François Hollande (the leader of the socialist party) have been together for years, have four children together but never married. I ask her if this was a conscious decision. She laughs, 'No, it was more a question of finding the time,' she says. 'And we both use our own names so it would have complicated things.'

So will we see President Chirac's demise coincide with the rise of Madame Royal? 'It's very flattering that people talk about me in that context,' she says. 'But it's not something I think about every day.' Unlike most of the rest of the nation. You can't pick up a newspaper without seeing her picture on the front of it.

Clara Gaymard is another example of a French superwoman. She is their answer to Nicola Horlick, the City banker and mother of six. She has not six but eight children aged between seven and seventeen. But where Horlick is perhaps best described as motherly, Gaymard is pencil thin and always well turned out, with a blonde bob and well-cut suits.

Clara concedes that she would not have been able to have eight children had she lived in England or America. She does not have a million pound banker's salary. 'I don't think I could have done what I have done if I hadn't lived in France,' she says. 'We have a lot of help in the system, we can deduct tax with each child, and there are no social charges for the staff we employ to look after them. The French system gives a woman the opportunity of being a mother and having a career.'

Edith Cresson, the former Prime Minister of France,

agrees with her. I meet Cresson at her office in the eighth district of Paris close to the Alma Bridge where she is now running the Second Chance Schools, a Europe-wide initiative for pupils who have failed the existing education system. It seems appropriate that she is running something called second chance; this is a woman who knows more about being given another chance than most people.

She is famous for gaffes. She once attributed the Japanese economic success to their 'ant-like' qualities. She contributed to the mass resignation of the European Commission in March 1999 when she was investigated for paying a dentist friend of hers almost $183,000 in consultancy fees. She had a short and unpopular reign as prime minister, lasting only ten months. At the time she blamed her downfall on a macho plot.

The woman Mitterrand referred to as 'my little soldier' greets me and asks me to sit down. She is not pretty, but I can imagine she was once attractive. Like most French women she is well groomed and very presentable. I find there is something of a lack of equilibrium in her face and wonder whether she has been secretly botoxing.

We begin with the question of working women. She tells me the French have got it right when it comes to supporting women who want to work and have children. 'It is not like Germany here where you are looked down upon if you go back to work. What works well here in France is family politics. In Germany women are choosing not to have children so they can continue to work.'

I can only agree with her. One of the main advantages I found when moving here was the childcare system. It really is geared to making life easier for mothers. I have a childminder who is subsidised by the state. Even if I didn't have her, all my children would be able to go the state primary school '*maternelle*' section from the age of two. This is of course free of charge. At school there is a crèche service so you can leave the children earlier in the morning if you need to and collect them later on. In addition, I pay less tax than I did in England because we have so many children.

Back to politics. I have yet to meet a female politician who hasn't been accused of having an affair with Mitterrand. I can only assume he was very good at multi-tasking. I don't quite know why I am so determined to ask Cresson the one question I have not dared ask the others, maybe because all the adverse publicity she has generated has lessened my respect for her. I know she is going to hate it, but here I go.

'There is a rumour,' I begin rather pathetically. 'That Mitterrand gave you the job as prime minister because you were having an affair. Is this true?'

'Do you really think the President of the Republic of France would choose his mistress as Prime Minister?' she fires back at me. Well, now you mention it, why not? France has a long history of royal mistresses ruling the nation.

'I was a minister five times before becoming prime minister, I was elected mayor of my town, and I was on the regional council. I have proved myself again and again politically. I find it stupefying that people still say I slept my way to the top,' she goes on.

She then tells me that two prime ministers were given the role without being elected and how unfair it is that no one questions how they got there, whereas she got there through a democratic process. 'Then the press says I have never denied it. Why should I?' Well, it might stop people speculating I'm tempted to say.

Cresson suffered the indignity of a right-wing MP shouting '*Voila La Pompadour*' (a reference to Louis XV's mistress) when she walked into the national assembly as prime minister for the first time. As if this wasn't bad enough, when she became agriculture minister she went to a demonstration of farmers who had written on a huge poster: '*Edith on t'espère meilleure au lit qu'au ministère*'— Edith we hope you're better in bed than as a minister.

The former Miss France, Sophie Tellier says this kind of sexism is not limited to politics. 'It doesn't matter what job a woman is in, if she gets anywhere she has automatically slept with someone,' she says. 'Especially if she's pretty, because then of course she is also viewed as stupid. Luckily I had studied law before I won Miss France; otherwise I would have been viewed as just a bimbo. In France women have to work twice as hard to prove themselves, it is a very macho society.'

Even a male friend of mine living and working in Paris confirms this. He works in a bank where one of the managing directors is female. 'The rumour is that she gives the CEO blow-jobs most days,' says Ed. 'But frankly I don't believe it, she just doesn't look the type. I certainly wouldn't want her giving me a blow-job.'

After my meeting with Edith Cresson I meet B for lunch in a bistro around the corner. He is waiting for me when I arrive. In this he is not typically French. I have never known people be so late as they are in France. Now when I arrange to meet French friends I ask them if they mean English time or French time. If they say French time I show up twenty minutes late and bring a book in case they're even later.

I immediately ask him about the beastly way the male politicians treat women. He of course defends himself and tells me that women are given a lot of breaks in politics, that there is positive discrimination and that male MPs are simply not allowed to go around being sexist. I also ask him if all these women did sleep with Mitterrand.

'You Brits have such hang ups about sex,' he tells me grinning broadly. 'In France we don't care who our politicians are sleeping with as long as they're doing a good job.'

I try to argue that maybe having someone give you a

blow-job who isn't your wife is a reflection on your character, or lack of it. B looks at me quizzically. 'Do you think giving someone a blow-job makes you a worse person?' Infuriatingly I start blushing.

'You should try to relax about sex,' he continues. 'In Italy they say you can't eat the same sauce with your pasta every day.'

'So do you often have a different sauce?' I ask. 'What does your wife think of that?' B sighs and puts down his knife and fork. A rare occurrence in itself for a French man between the hours of 12.30 and 1.30. 'You Anglo-Saxons are so brutally honest,' he says. 'Why do you have to tell everyone everything? What good does it do?' So like all good politicians he has failed to answer my question.

After lunch I walk to the Faubourg Saint-Honoré where I meet Inès de la Fressange for a coffee. I ask her if she finds it tough juggling her career and family life. 'I have decided it's impossible,' she tells me with her characteristic candour. 'In magazines you read about these perfect women who live in complete order and drink a glass of water before even getting out of bed. They have everything organised from nannies to menus, everything seems fantastic. I have decided that if you're a mother and working you're going to feel guilty wherever you are. Either in the office when the phone rings and there's some problem at school, or at home when you feel you should be in the office. You just have to accept that you're not going to be the perfect woman,' she says looking incredibly perfect. So what does she do? 'Accept that you may not be the perfect mother, but that your children can't find a better one and they're very happy with you. Accept that things can be a bit messy and it's not a disaster if the bed isn't made. Accept that you're not five different people at once and just relax a bit. Think about your priorities too. Is it more important to stay in the office or to go home to my children?'

Sophie Sarkozy says the key to a successful career and home life is organisation and delegation. 'It is easy to combine the two,' she tells me. 'You just need someone at home who is the oil of the engine. I have decided I can't let having both a career and family life be a problem so I pay someone a lot of money to be at home and do all the things I can't do such as cooking, shopping, looking after the children. I also have a company that looks after my car. The trick is to pay luxury companies to organise your life, if you try to do it all yourself it's hell.' Good advice, but I get the impression Sophie lives on a slightly different economic level to the rest of us. This is a woman who has a personal trainer and twice-weekly massages.

The female politicians I spoke to told me there is a great solidarity between French women at work. 'The men are not all macho,' says Anne Hidalgo at the Paris mayor's office. 'But some of them are inclined to follow their instincts. If you are attacked in a sexist manner, there will be support from both left and right.' Cresson says this was the case when she was called *La Pompadour*. The offending politician's secretary threatened to resign over it.

But it seems this solidarity is not the same in the private sector. My friend Simon who is married to a French woman says his wife has turned down two jobs which meant she would be working for a woman. 'They are very unkind to their fellow women,' he says. 'My wife now says she doesn't want to work for a woman or even employ one.' Sophie Tellier agrees. 'I prefer to work with men because I find the perpetual comparisons between women exhausting.'

I can't say what they are like to work with an office environment. The only other living creature in my office is normally Max the cat. But I can imagine it must be quite tough. French women are already competitive when it comes to men, looks, clothes and handbags. Put a career on top of that and you end up with a potentially lethal combination.

9

Le Bébé surprise

'There is nothing inherently creative about giving birth.'
Simone de Beauvoir

One of the first things I did when we moved to France was have a baby. I was already seven months pregnant when we left England, a slightly mad state to be in for a major life change. My first memories of my new life in France are of unpacking boxes and planning the delivery of our second child.

To the French I was a mystery. First of all I had no idea of the sex of my baby, nor did I want to know. 'Aahh,' my obstetrician would say every time I went to see him. '*Le bébé surprise.*'

In France most women find out the sex of their baby as early as possible. 'I think it's ridiculous not to find out,' says Hermine de Clermont-Tonnerre, who is pregnant with her second child, and due to find out the sex a week later. 'I like a surprise when it's a beautiful present, but not when it's my baby. This way I can organise everything.'

When I was pregnant with my third child, I was praying for a boy. I had even done a boy diet based on red wine and meat—so not really a hardship—and got into all sorts of strange positions to conceive. It was my husband's one criterion for allowing me to have the baby. His last three had been girls and a fourth would have been too much, he said. He had a friend at school who had four sisters. Every time he opened a cupboard a box of tampons fell on his head. This was not a fate my husband was willing to share. I decided not to find out the sex. I figured if a girl, I would have had to listen to my husband complaining for the next six months, which would just be too hateful.

A few days after my amniocentesis, I came home to a message on the answer machine. It was my obstetrician's secretary. 'Hello Madame,' she began. 'Just to let you know the results of your amniocentesis are in and they're all fine and it is a ...' at this stage I wondered whether to hang up and not listen any more. My whole body froze. Of course I did carry on listening: 'a little boy.'

I immediately burst into tears much to the amazement of a friend who was staying at the time. 'But isn't that what you wanted?' he asked. Of course it was, and I was crying from relief, but also about the fact that the magical moment when the baby comes out and the surprise of that had been taken away. The only French woman I know who has not known the sex of her baby in advance is my friend Alexandra.

Another reason I was a mystery to the medical establishment at my hospital was that I wanted a natural birth. During the birth of our first baby I had been immersed in a birthing pool with nothing but oxygen to help me along. It hurt like hell but I felt great afterwards and I was keen to repeat the experience.

Ask any French woman if they would consider childbirth without drugs and they look at you as if you just suggested they give up baguettes or nail varnish. 'Why?' is the most common response. 'Are you mad?' often follows. So it was with my handsome obstetrician. Shaking his head, he sent me off to see the anaesthetist so that if I needed one, I could have an epidural. As it turned out, Beatrice was a breach baby and delivered by caesarean section: so much for all my forward planning.

Once installed in my single room with TV in the clinic where I had Beatrice I noticed that the use of painkillers and the accommodation were not the only thing that differed in France. Most of the mothers on my ward were bottle feeding.

Back at the natural birthing centre in Crowborough,

Sussex, they practically won't allow you in unless you promise to breastfeed. In some countries, like Sweden and Australia, bottle-feeding a new born is akin to some minor crimes, in fact some major ones. In Australia women regularly breastfeed for a year. I was desperate to talk to these French women and tell them they were depriving their babies of the best possible start in life. At the time I spoke about seven words of French (three of them being *par le siège*—breach) so I couldn't begin to formulate a convincing argument.

My English friend Jeanette has had both her babies here. She is astounded by the French attitude to childbearing and child-rearing. 'There seem to be two main desirables in France,' she says. 'One is not to have a fat tummy when pregnant; you have to put on twenty pounds, no more. The second is how to get a child to have no need for you at all once it's born.'

This is one of the reasons a lot of French women don't breastfeed. Only two per cent of the women I interviewed had breastfed. Official statistics put the figure higher. In 2002, fifty six per cent breastfed compared to a figure in the UK of sixty nine per cent. But I have a suspicion the French statistic includes women like one I spoke to in Paris who said her hospital was very pro-breastfeeding, so she did it for the three days she was there and then stopped as soon as she got home.

'You're a freak if you breastfeed here,' says Jeanette. 'I

had two babies and they gave them both the bottle without even asking me. With the first one I didn't even see her for three days as she was in an incubator.' When she was reunited with her daughter, Jeanette started to breastfeed her, ignorant of the fact that the medicines they were giving her for high blood pressure were highly dangerous for the baby. The baby then started having heart problems. 'I had to pump out milk so my supply didn't dry up and throw it away for two weeks until the medicine had gone through my system,' she says. 'Then I had to teach my daughter to breastfeed all over again. I really felt it was me against the system.'

Jeanette thinks this aversion to breastfeeding is rooted in the French woman's desire to be constantly seductive. 'Here you have to be sexy or you're dead,' she says. 'If you're not, then you're worse than invisible, a nuisance taking up space on the sidewalk. The only way to get across a zebra crossing is to show your cleavage.'

A French woman I met at a party told me she hadn't breastfed because her breasts were for her husband. I felt like bashing her on the head with a basic biology manual. Maybe they are all influenced by Simone de Beauvoir who said that giving birth is all about being weighed down, and that it drags women back into the animal realm and away from creative fulfilment. Needless to say de Beauvoir couldn't—or wouldn't—have children.

French women are obsessed with the way they look, so

anything that might make your breasts sag is a no-no. They also don't like all that messy milk staining their expensive clothes. Added to which having to get your breasts out in public makes your choice of what to wear so limited. But more than anything they don't like to be tied down, they don't like their *liberté* messed with.

In the town near where I live there are several underwear shops. My favourite one is run by a beautiful woman who just had a baby. In fact before she had the baby I remember asking her when it was due. She was tiny so I assumed she was around five months pregnant. 'Any day now,' she told me. She had the baby and three weeks later was back at work looking pencil thin and stunning again. It was actually quite scary.

'Aren't you breastfeeding?' was of course my first question.

'Oh no,' she said. 'She's quite happy with a bottle.'

It wasn't only the fact that she wasn't breastfeeding that upset me. It was the fact that she looked so damned perfect, so soon after having a baby, almost like the baby had never happened. Whatever happened to blobbing around with your newborn, enjoying those first few weeks, getting to know the little person you've just given birth to?

But as Naomi Wolf observes, French women do not let children or childbirth get in the way of looking good. 'I find it hard to be on holiday without deconstructing gender norms between the French and American women. The

French had a way of walking around in their bikinis with an innate coquettish charm. Most of the Americans have parked that part of themselves in a box when they get married and have children. I had to admire the way the French women could lie in the sun, so nonchalantly topless, while all these very sturdy beach boys brought them towels. They certainly know how to fly the flag of their sex.'

One of the French women I spoke to excused the fact that she didn't breastfeed saying she had hired a maternity nurse and it just wasn't worth having a dog and barking yourself. She told me she had to hire a maternity nurse so that she could still go out for dinner with her husband while the baby was small. 'I want things to stay just as they always have been,' she told me.

This might come as a surprise, but things do change when you have a baby. I can understand the desire not to alienate your husband by spending the first three months wrapped up in baby feeding and so on, but it is such a short time and so important for the child that you would think most women would just do it automatically. You've got the rest of your life to go out to dinner. (And if your breasts do sag as a result of breastfeeding, in France you can get a boob-job on the national health plan.)

You also get pelvic re-education on the national health. This is an extraordinary experience and one that should not be missed. It is worth having children here just to go through it. Apart from any benefits to your sex life and future incontinence levels, it means you will be immune to embarrassment for the rest of your life because nothing can ever be as bad as this.

A few months after the birth of my third child, I go along to my local *kiné*, a good-looking man in his thirties called Nicolas. *Kinés* are a very French thing; a mixture between osteopaths and masseurs. Nicolas tells me to take my trousers and underwear off. Then he tells me to lie down on a couch with my legs apart. At this moment I am asking myself if I will ever recover. Then it gets worse. Nicolas pulls on a white diaphanous plastic glove and smears his two forefingers with gel. I am now starting to perspire. 'This is not happening,' I think. I close my eyes and pray that it is a bad dream. It's not. 'Squeeze please,' he tells me as calmly as if he were ordering a bag of chips. I do as I'm told. 'Hmm, not bad for three children,' he says. 'Sometimes they squeeze and I can't feel a thing.' I take this as a compliment but say nothing as I am finding it impossible to speak.

This preliminary session is the first of twenty. The rest of them will involve the marginally less embarrassing ritual of placing something that looks like a cross between a vibrator and an instrument of torture inside me. This is attached to a box which gives me small electric shocks and a pattern on a screen I have to follow by squeezing. Who knows if it's made any difference, but it was one of those things I had to try.

The refusal of French women to breastfeed is such a contradiction as I have never met a race more obsessed with child health, safety and nutrition. I remember one evening I was cooking dinner for the girls. It was the standard thing any British mother might feed them; chicken nuggets and chips. My friend Alexandra was visiting and horrified.

'I can't believe how healthily you eat compared to the rubbish you feed your children,' she said. This is a woman who I have seen knock up three exquisite meals for one dinner. One for Elisa, another for the baby Astrid and a third for her and Jean-Claude. All of the meals will consist of fresh vegetables and meat or fish. Since that day I haven't bought another chicken nugget or chip. When she came round the other night, I was about to feed the children gnocchi and a shop-bought sauce. I quickly hid the sauce at the back of the cupboard and started knocking up a fresh tomato one instead. In fact, I found that once you start cooking proper food for them, it really doesn't take that much more time. Quite apart from being amazed by the things they will eat—like asparagus, artichokes, oysters and *saucisson*—I rather like the saintly glow I feel as I serve them a home-cooked dinner. Not a feeling I am terribly used to.

In France family mealtimes are sacred. A year after we moved in, Jean-François, the electrician, was fixing the spotlights in the kitchen. I was feeding Olivia (then aged one) and Bea who was a few months old. He asked me why I wasn't eating at the same time. 'My husband and I eat together later on,' I told him.

He was horrified. Eating together as a family is an essential part of growing up for the children, he told me. How will they ever learn to eat properly if we don't eat with them? What will it do for our relationship with them if we exclude them from our meals?

I wanted to protest and say that nothing could be as bad as trying to enjoy one's dinner while Bea stuffed *petits pois* up her nose, but decided to smile benignly and mutter something about cultural differences. But now when I go back to England, I am shocked at how much worse the children behave at the table. OK, mine are pretty bad, as I said to Agnès at Tiffany's, I'm always having to tell them to sit down. She looked at me sympathetically and said she has the impression she is always telling her children not to talk with their mouth full, don't put your elbows on the table etc.

'But,' she added—in an off-hand way only a French woman could—'telling them to sit down, that would be a bit basic.'

I noted with some joy a few weekends ago in a beach restaurant that Olivia started mass dissent in the French children's camp. Of course they were all sitting down being perfectly behaved. But Olivia was tearing around. Gradually one joined, then another, then another. It was like watching soldiers gradually deserting from an army. The parents got up and shouted at them at first but after a while even they gave up.

Because the children often come home from school for lunch, you get to shout at them for three meals a day and not just two. In fact making the children eat in the canteen at school is seen as a form of punishment, according to a friend of mine in the village.

I can't quite see how a four-course lunch can be seen as punishment. I have been amazed by the quality of food here. The lunch menus in France in both primary and secondary schools will always include a starter, a main course of meat or fish with vegetables, a dairy product and a dessert. In some schools they have a self-service system with a range of colours for food: one colour for vegetables, another one for milk products, another for meat and so on. Pupils need to take one dish of each colour, to make sure they have a balanced diet. Although they don't have this in my children's school, they try to influence them to eat up or try at least everything that is on their plate.

Some friends of mine called Sarah and Andrew moved to the Gers two years ago with their ten-year-old son Thomas. 'Back in English school he was eating pizzas three times a week,' says Sarah.

The kinds of food Thomas now eats include asparagus quiche, tuna and egg salad, soup or savoury filled pancake. Main courses are usually duck, chicken, pork or fish accompanied by rice, potatoes or pasta and at least one vegetable. The desserts are yogurt or *fromage blanc* with fruit or sugar.

'What I love here is that the kids grow up learning to try everything,' says Sarah. 'Thomas would never have touched a lentil at home and now he asks if we can have lentils and sausages for dinner.' At Thomas's school the food is sourced locally by the dinner lady. 'Some of the vegetables even come from her garden,' says Sarah. 'But we are talking a very little school.'

The whole country stops at 12 o'clock so the French can enjoy the sacred hour of the *déjeuner*. (Where we are in the south it usually runs into two sacred hours and then a siesta.) The healthy eating habits of the French must come from somewhere. Maybe a school dinner of three or four courses is where they begin?

Not only do the French eat in with their children, they eat out with them too. During the summer in a village close to here they have a party every Friday evening. It is one of the best knees-up I have ever been to. The whole village is there, with ages ranging from new-born to nudging ninety and beyond.

Vast tables are laid out under the plane trees in the main square with white paper cloths on them. There is seating for around two hundred people. At the end of the tables three huge bonfires burn, ready for the spit-roast which is either wild boar or pig. For $18 per adult and $5 per child you will be given as much pastis, water and wine as you can drink and a four-course dinner. The only thing you need to bring is plates, knives and forks and nibbles for the aperitif. The children all run around all evening (apart from when they're eating obviously, and then it's only my children who are running around).

The wonderful thing is not only that the adults mix with the children but that the children of all ages play together. There is a dance after dinner and you will see toddlers dancing with teenagers, as well as grandparents.

The French are much more inclusive of children as a rule. They put up with them being around more than the English do. You can walk into any restaurant here with children and know they will be welcomed.

In the five years we have been here, we have never been stared at for taking our children anywhere. People actively help you with your children, they stop you in the street to chat with them; strangers give them little presents. French women, especially the older ones, seem unable to keep their hands off children, they love patting their heads. Maybe it is part of the kissing thing; people are so much more tactile here. Tony, a friend who has lived here for fifteen years, says one of the most amazing things he has ever seen is his teenage daughter getting on a school bus and kissing everyone on it as she makes her way to her seat. When we go to dinner with French friends here, their children (even if they have never met us) will come up and kiss us hello. It all seems incredibly civilised.

The downside is a huge measure of control. When we went to the local primary school to see the headmistress and register our children, she was in the middle of teaching a class. She came out into the corridor to speak to us and as far as I could make out the children were being very quiet. After a couple of minutes she excused herself and went back into the classroom. She shouted at the class, telling them to be quiet and do as they'd been told. Delighted as I was at the prospect of this woman taking charge of my wild girls, I did wonder what on earth she would do if they were really bad. I have seen children being physically punished more here than in England.

Parents also seem to want to be in control within an inch. We were on the beach the other day and the ice-cream man came along. Our girls and some girls they had been playing with ran up to him. I went to buy them an ice-cream and asked the mother of the other children if I could buy them one. 'No,' she said. 'It's not tea-time.' In fact it was half past three, so not a million miles away from tea-time. Her children were of course heartbroken and had to watch mine smugly stuffing themselves with ice-lollies. This control seems part of the overall French psyche. The women are in control of themselves, their bodies, the way they look, they watch their diet, and every element of their lives. Their children are just another thing they want to control.

There is no doubt they are stricter with their children here than we are in England and the US. There are certain rules that are kept to and manners that are obligatory. The only thing they don't do is the very English 'thank you for my dinner please may I get down'. I find my children can be as badly behaved as they like but if they do this the French are incredibly impressed and will mutter on for ever about how '*bien élevé*' they are.

Hermine de Clermont-Tonnerre told me she thought manners and a love of life were the most important things to pass on to one's children. (I must point out here though that Hermine, charming as she is, showed up late and also failed to thank me for tea.) Manners do figure highly in French society. It is altogether more formal than English society.

The nanny state starts at birth here. It is one of the major contradictions of France. They are so mad about freedom, but they dictate everything you do. You have the freedom to go on holiday—as long as it is in August. You can go on holiday anywhere you like—as long as it's in France. You are told by a paediatrician when you can start feeding your child solids. And if you have a French mother, you will be protected from every eventuality by her. My friend Emmanuelle, who has two girls, drives me totally insane at times. They come here to play. We have a lovely garden, swimming pool, a hammock, swings and things to climb on. If one of the girls so much as sniffs, she's not allowed in the pool, which of course means she spends the whole day weeping and watching the others frolicking about. They are not allowed to take their shoes off and run around the garden in case they stand on something. They're not allowed to climb on the swings in case they fall down. If it's sunny, they have to wear a hat. And sun cream and a T-shirt to protect their shoulders. She spends more time fussing about, than actually enjoying what she came here for; the open space and freedom to do what they want as they're not cooped up in their town house for once. I asked her why she didn't just let them get on with it.

'It's all right for you,' she snapped back. 'Your children are never ill.'

That's probably because I expose them to the odd germ or bit of cold I felt like telling her. But of course I don't. French women seem to have a real thing about children getting cold. Chantal, my childminder, comes and collects the children in the morning. In the summer it is already hot by 8.30 am and they are skipping about in shorts and T-shirts.

'I think they might need *un petit pull*' (a pullover), she says, eyeing the sky suspiciously although the sun is so bright one can hardly venture out without at least two pairs of sun glasses on and there isn't a cloud to be seen. In the winter (and the winters here are not what one would call arctic) you will see children stuffed into prams with so many clothes on they can hardly breathe. All you can see of them is this little face half-covered in hat and scarf. I'm sure hundreds grow up with severe claustrophobia. Jeanette, my Montpellier friend, says people actually stop her in the street in the winter to tell her that her children aren't sufficiently clothed. She also gets into trouble on the beach. Her girls, aged six and three, will never keep their hats on. A woman once went up to her and started giving her a lecture about the dangers of sun-burn. 'I felt like asking what she suggested I do, super-glue the hats to their skulls?' she says.

Another difference is the way in which little girls behave. They are somehow more flirtatious and feminine than English girls. A story the Irish writer Norrie Hearn once told me confirms this. When I explained to him that I was writing a book trying to define and understand French chic, he told me about a young exchange student he once had to stay with him when he was living in Somerset. 'Christelle, a nine year old, stayed with us simply because her age matched one of our daughters,' he said. 'I was amazed every morning when this little girl prepared for school. On would go her trousers and a shirt and then she'd pick up a scarf, toss it round her neck, run a comb through her hair—and she looked, well, *chic*. She made the village kids look like clodhoppers and without any apparent effort. Is it genetic?'

During my research I was intrigued to find out if it was true that French women instinctively know how to tie a scarf. I asked my publishing friend Charlotte.

'No,' she said. 'I don't think so.' She got her scarf and put it on in a way I have never seen an English woman put a scarf on. She started at the front and then came back over her shoulders with the ends. The result was extremely elegant.

I think there are good things to be learnt from the way French women bring up their children; the discipline, the eating, the way they dress them and the way they include them at mealtimes are all great. But I long to tell them just to relax, that there is no evidence that not wearing a scarf, hat and gloves when it's sixty degrees outside leads directly to fatal pneumonia.

Some friends of ours who live in the Dordogne are always arguing about the children and the way they should be raised. It is one of the clearest examples of cultural differences I have seen. She is French and he is English. They have two sons. He wants to send them to boarding school in England, she won't even hear of it. In France boarding school is not a luxury, but seen as a punishment. 'It's just impossible,' says the husband. 'Trying to get a French mother to part with her sons is like trying to get the pope to convert to Lutheranism. There is just no way, although I think they would benefit hugely from exposure to the two cultures (and also from some time away from an over-protective mother).'

As things are, our children will grow up to be more French than anything else. Does that matter? I was very worried when we first moved here that I wouldn't be able to relate to them, that they wouldn't understand the jokes in *Fawlty Towers* for example. It seems a little less important now. The girls still speak English to each other and I am hoping that they always will (at least I'll be able to understand them).

But the other day Bea and I had a rather worrying exchange. She told me she hated our family, which was 'boring' and that she wanted to go and live with my childminder Chantal's family. I asked her why. She said something completely incomprehensible which I didn't recognise as French but guess it must have been. I asked her to repeat it several times but still couldn't understand.

'There, you see,' she said throwing down her school bag in irritation. 'That's why I want to leave; you never understand anything I say.'

And she's only five.

10

Ten Kilos

'Elegance is refusal.'
Coco Chanel

I have an English male friend living in Paris who is a philanderer. I don't know many of them, but Christopher is very active on the pulling front. The last time I had a drink with him he received four messages on his mobile phone from different women in half an hour. One from his girlfriend (poor love), another from an English girl he had slept with two nights before, another from a French girl he had slept with that morning and the fourth from another French girl he was planning to sleep with once he'd finished his whisky.

As he is such an expert on women I asked him what the

difference is between French women and English women.

'About ten kilos' (twenty-two pounds), he replied.

There is no denying it. French women are thinner than us. By a long shot. On my last visit home I saw more fat people in an hour at the Eurostar terminal than I had done during a five-day visit to Paris.

When I moved here, I was seven months pregnant so there really wasn't much I could do about my weight. But a few months after our daughter Beatrice was born, I started to think about dieting so that I could stop wearing maternity clothes and feeling like I would never fit into a normal pair of trousers again. I was also horribly aware that I was by far the fattest person I knew. The strange thing is that if everyone around you is thin, it makes you want to be thin too.

So motivation to lose weight was easy, now I just had to work our how to do it. I was still eating and drinking very much like an English girl. In fact, so as not to deprive myself, I had travelled to France with several bottles of my favourite Chardonnay. Once I had drunk the last of these, I wondered whether it was time to go native.

I decide to consult Inès de la Fressange, as she is the thinnest woman I know. When I meet her for advice, she is in an exceptionally good mood. I wonder if perhaps her daughter, a judo enthusiast, has made it to black belt. Or if the brand she is busy reviving, Roger Vivier shoes, has been picked up by *Vogue* as the season's must-have accessory.

No, this is much bigger news: 'They're finally stocking Crunchie bars at the Bon Marché,' she tells me smiling broadly. 'I just love them and used to cram my pockets full of them at Heathrow, but now that I don't travel to London very often, I don't get the opportunity.'

This is the kind of statement that makes the rest of the world's female population hate French women. How, we ask, is it possible to eat Crunchie bars and still look like a waif?

In fact, let's look at the list of foods on your average French woman's diet sheet: *foie gras* (nice and slimming, especially with a little bit of sugar-rich onion or fig pickle to go with it), cheese (we're talking full-fat get a load of this oozing, creamy stuff here, not half-fat Philadelphia), croissants (and to really add insult to injury, they sometimes put butter and jam on top). The list goes on. So how does she do it?

'I simply stop eating when I'm not hungry,' says Inès. 'For me hunger comes only from my stomach, I am not one of those people who eats for comfort. If I want to feel good I go shopping for something exceptional to treat myself.'

I think this is the key. French women eat small portions. They don't overindulge when it comes to bits of baguette that are ruthlessly thrown in their general direction several times a day. The French actress Elisabeth Bourgine sums up their mentality. 'I don't diet,' she says. 'I adore gourmand food but I am careful and there is no overindulgence.'

All You Need to Be Impossibly French

All French women say they watch what they eat. 'I haven't had a croissant in ten years,' says Agnès Cromback from Tiffany's. Anny Duperey, for example, says she eats porridge in the morning and when she's at home she is extremely careful, eating mainly steamed fish and vegetables. 'But when I go out, I eat exactly what I want,' she says. Some French women take this a step further. My friend Simon has been living in Paris for nineteen years and is married to Isabelle, an extremely thin French woman. 'When we go out, she'll often eat more than I do,' he explains. 'But that will probably be the only decent meal she's had in two days. I never see her eat breakfast.'

Sophie Sarkozy says she is always careful about what she eats. She works in PR and so lunches with clients a lot. 'Sometimes I have the restaurant prepare just a plate of exotic fruit,' she says. 'The only difficult thing about diet is presentation. Of course if you sit down in front of the TV with a low-fat yoghurt and a banana, it's depressing, but if you have a chef prepare a fantastic picture from fruit, it looks appetising.' Sophie says that if she eats out too much for one day over the weekend say, she will then be exceptionally careful for two days. 'I was told by a doctor that you need two days of attention for one day of letting yourself go,' she says.

It is but a small change in how you think. I am quite able to munch my way through an entire slab of brie, but have learnt to control myself. Every time I am about to go for that third helping, I think about my new jeans. They are devastating but slightly tight—I was told by a French shop assistant that I must on no account buy a size twelve if I can squeeze into a ten.

Gradually I did begin to lose weight again. But it wasn't just willpower that was helping me. It was something else, something much more fundamental. Lingerie designer Chantal Thomass has a factory in Nottingham where she produces a range of underwear destined for the US. She spends several weeks a year there and says that she never fails to put on weight during that time. She blames this on the sandwiches she had for lunch. 'There is no other choice, you eat so badly over there' she says. 'I come back to Paris and have to diet; basically I just don't eat much for a few days.'

France is a just a very good place to lose weight. In the early 1990s scientists noted the French paradox that despite the fact that the French eat masses of runny cheeses, kilos of pâté and *foie gras*, drink gallons of wine and smoke millions of cigarettes, they are thirty per cent less likely to die from heart disease than their counterparts in the US or northern Europe. They also noted that the southern French were thirty per cent less likely to suffer from heart conditions than the northern French. The French diet is not just beneficial for the heart but also leads to less bowel cancer, fewer circulatory problems, less osteoporosis and other problems. In fact a recent study showed that men that had already suffered a heart attack and switched to a more Mediterranean based diet cut their chances of a second heart attack by almost seventy per cent.

Brigitte Papin, Health and Beauty editor of *Madame Figaro* magazine, says it is the French culture of eating that helps them to stay thin. 'We don't eat that terrible fattening white bread you have or drink milk until we're teenagers,' she says. According to Dr Bouget, a nutritionist at the Bichat Hospital in Paris, the difference in diets between French and English women goes back to the industrial revolution. 'The English working in the factories quickly lost touch with fundamentals such as fruit, and vegetables that are so central to the French diet even today,' he says. 'England changed its habits very quickly and became a fast-food nation, eating chips and drinking too much alcohol.'

My diet certainly has changed from living in France. There is still the tradition here of shopping for the day, so you tend to come back with fresh produce that you prepare and eat on the day you buy it. There are markets in most villages, oyster cabins in our local town where you can pick up a dozen opened oysters for next to nothing and lots of options for healthy eating. In the summer you can throw together a lunch made up of tomatoes, bread, olive oil and cheese which can taste glorious. This means you are not eating pre-packaged foods which are in the main unhealthy and fattening. They also don't satisfy you as much as fresh food does so you stay hungry.

So are French women thinner because they live in France or because of something that culturally keeps them on the straight and narrow, or because of some other secret? All the fresh food you need is readily available everywhere, so you can't use not living near the Mediterranean as an excuse not to eat well. It is a diet that is easy to follow wherever you are. Essentially it means choosing fish above red meat, olive oil at every given opportunity, and having at least two glasses of red wine a day. Hardly a hardship. (And if you're worried about wine being fattening, don't. A bottle of Languedoc red is 680 calories, the equivalent of a cheeseburger and chips, and probably better for you.)

And where are the French who indulge in all the bad processed foods in life? A lot of the chic Parisians I meet tell me they never snack. They are so thin I begin to think most of them wouldn't recognise a crisp if it came and hit them in the face. They never eat them, they tell me. Just the word 'crisp' makes them go slightly pale.

I believed them until I went to the offices of a major Paris fashion magazine that shall remain nameless to protect its reputation. Of course I have the usual crisis about what to wear, how my hair looks and most importantly how I can look my absolute thinnest. For lunch I have a minimal amount of sushi (how many fat Japanese women do you know?), a green tea and then I go for a long walk before showing up at the appointed hour of two o'clock.

I am greeted by two female journalists who are both extremely senior writers for the magazine. They are not thin. That is the first total shock. There is worse to come. One of them is carrying a half-eaten box of small pretzel-style snacks which she is merrily tucking into. My jaw is now closer to the floor than my upper lip. The other one, oh my God could it get any worse?—is actually drinking a Coke. And what's more even offers me one. I am stunned.

'So, as you can see,' laughs one of them settling into a sofa clutching her pretzels. 'We don't get fat.' I smile politely and try to regain my composure—all my images of perfect Parisians shattered.

Another thing that shocks me is how much French women smoke. Go into any bar in Paris and the stench of tobacco floors you. Sylvaine Ratte, tobacco programme director of France's cancer society, admits that the ban on smoking in restaurants and cafés in Paris has been a total failure. 'It was a disaster,' she says. 'People just ignored it.'

According to an article in the *New York Times* by journalism lecturer Jessica Seigel, in France smoking is much more prevalent among those on a higher income than it is in the United States. There only one in ten of those on a high income smoke, in France it is one in three. Catherine Deneuve, arguably the most iconic of French women, second only to the Statue of Liberty in New York, smokes. She gave up her sixty-a-day habit in the 1980s, only to find she put on weight and felt very un-French. In France smoking is linked to existentialist conversations in Parisian cafés. Deneuve once told a *Washington Post* reporter: 'A cigarette helps you think, you know.' She has started smoking again. As my French friend Sylvie sums up: 'Everyone smokes in France, it's just a question of how much.'

In fact obesity is on the rise in France. According to official statistics only six per cent of the French population was obese in 1990, but that has risen to eleven per cent today. In the US the figure is twenty two per cent and in the UK it is seventeen per cent for men and twenty one per cent of women. But an astounding fifty per cent of the UK population is classified as overweight. A book recently published by a French doctor called *Obesity—The New French Illness* claims that 19.8 million French people are overweight, and one in three is a woman.

It is hard interpret these figures, though. I was sitting outside a restaurant in Sète the other day and a truly fat French woman walked past. She was of Michelin-man proportions, all dressed in white. Not a good colour for the clinically obese. But what was more shocking was that we noticed. The friends we were with, who live in London, said in England it would be the other way round. You would notice a woman because she is thin.

Nonetheless, only fourteen per cent of French women say they feel good about their bodies according to the French National Scientific Research Centre, even though sixty one per cent weigh around the healthy norm. As Brigitte Papin says: 'All French women, without exception, will always say they have five pounds to lose. Our most popular articles are always about wrinkles or slimming.'

French women may not do the Atkins diet (I mean, really, can you imagine a French woman not eating bread or cheese?) but they have other methods to help them when temptation has got the better of them.

There are a lot of closely guarded secrets lurking in the French pharmacy. There they sell all sorts of 'healthy' diet aids. These range from phials of strange looking liquid to pills that eliminate water retention to pastilles you chew.

I have tried some of them and they may work for the French, but not being a masochist willing to suffer for the sake of slimming I remain unimpressed. There is one particularly unpleasant mixture of squashed up figs: you have it an hour before your meal and drink lots of water. This indigestible concoction then expands in your stomach and sends a signal to your brain telling it you're not hungry. It certainly put me off eating but mainly because it stuck my jaws together so that I was unable chew anything at all.

Another one I tried was a mix of green tea, ginseng and elderflower, also meant to reduce your appetite. The idea is to drink it first thing in the morning after you have mixed the contents with some water. As a device for waking you up it's great. A more foul-tasting thing you could not wish for, it really sharpens your senses. I don't think it made any difference in how much I ate, but as it is so disgusting it certainly put me off breakfast. Another magical bottle, this one a lurid purple, calls itself *Minceur Express* (slimming express). You mix it with one and a half litres of water a day and sip periodically. The effect of drinking so much water meant I felt more satiated than normal but I also felt like a walking water bed. The best one I tried was, surprisingly, a homeopathic diet pill which you take half an hour before you eat and which suppresses your appetite. But I kept forgetting to take it half an hour before meals, so gave up in the end.

One of my French friends, Marie-Françoise from Pau, says she never uses her pharmacy if she wants to diet. Instead she and her husband simply don't eat an evening meal. 'We will have a yogurt and a piece of fruit in front of the television but that's it,' she says. 'You don't digest the food you eat in the evening so it's a bad time to eat. My other tip is to take time when eating, eat for pleasure, and not like a dog.'

I once skipped an evening meal when I spent the night in hospital with my daughter Bea. I felt really great the next day, much more awake and energetic than normal. I think the mini-fast is a good idea and I vowed to do it once a week. Needless to say I haven't yet done it. But I do sometimes manage a mini-detox. You just have fruit or vegetables for dinner, maybe asparagus followed by chopped-up fruit. You could also try a mini-fast which means eating normally until midday and then not eating again until the following morning. You shouldn't then overdose on bacon and eggs; rather take it easy with some hot water and lemon followed by fruit for breakfast and maybe some wholemeal bread.

If they do diet, they don't let on. One French trick I was told by Agnès is the following: 'I have seen lots of women ooh and aah over how good the food is, poke it about on their plate and not actually eat more than a couple of mouthfuls.' This is anti-social; in fact any sort of diet you embark on should be carried out alone. There is nothing more irritating than going out to dinner with someone who eats a salad leaf and nothing else. The point about the French mentality is that you don't need to resort to that kind of behaviour, but you do need to become aware of what you're eating.

In France they eat their greens. Women don't just eat a green salad with their food, but they eat it as a course in itself. I have often seen them order a small green salad instead of a starter in a restaurant. If they're feeling reckless and carefree, they may go for some parmesan shavings on top. We English might scoff at such a healthy option, but done properly, with a bit of rocket for added flavour, it's delicious and actually has you leaving the lunch table feeling thinner than when you sat down.

In fact, I become so obsessed with asparagus once the season starts that I eat them almost every day. It is the most amazing food, healthy, virtually calorie free depending on what you put on it, versatile and cheap (at least it is here). In the village next door to ours there is a young couple that sells them every evening between five and seven o'clock, lending a whole new meaning to the famous French *cinq à sept* (traditionally the time for adultery). They sell them in what they call *bottes* or bunches. Thick, fresh, green clumps of delicious asparagus for a couple of pounds. I pick them up on the way back from the school run, a sort of asparagus drive-thru.

There is no mystery to staying thin; it is basically a question of common sense and willpower. The French gastronome Brillat-Savarin in his *Physiology of Taste* published in 1825 said: 'Tell me what you eat and I will tell you what you are.' He also said: 'The destiny of nations depends on how they nourish themselves.'

The French have a long history of looking after themselves through their diet. To many of them it is second nature. But it's not rocket science.

If you get up in the morning and have a glass of hot water with some lemon followed by some fresh fruit and then a piece of toast as opposed to a fried bacon buttie and a coke, you're going to give yourself a better start to the day and a better chance of getting into your trousers. And buying fruit is no more difficult than buying bacon. For lunch in the winter I eat mostly soups and in the summer mostly salads. This makes me sound like a real swot, but I also eat industrial quantities of pasta. There is no reason salads need to be boring, you can put all sorts of things in them to spice them up. For example some melted goat's cheese on bits of baguette and a dressing made with olive oil and honey. The sweetness of the honey and the sharpness of the goat's cheese is a wonderful contrast.

I ask my friend Carla what she thinks of this French approach to eating. 'I'm all for the French method,' she says. 'But you haven't even mentioned my exclusive *foie gras* and white wine diet.' Carla's 'exclusive' diet involves eating nothing but *foie gras* and drinking litres of white wine; not very slimming but very good fun. She has an unexpected French ally, I discover.

France's most glamorous newsreader, Laurence Ferrari, likes nothing more than tucking into *foie gras* and spaghetti carbonara. She says that spaghetti carbonara is her 'favourite food'. This takes some believing as she is a woman so thin and elegant that it is hard to imagine her delicately nibbling on anything more substantial than a bowl of bean sprouts. The news that she likes a high cholesterol diet of bacon, eggs and pasta is more shocking than many of the scandals she reports. I now watch her on the lunchtime news to improve my French and, more importantly, to encourage me not to eat too much.

Is Madame Ferrari a freak of nature? When I first moved here, I was a bit like a kid in a sweet shop, trying everything in sight. I soon realised that wasn't the French way. As with their underwear, they go for quality and not quantity when they're eating. If you have a sweet tooth, it is easier to follow their lead and stock up with seriously sexy dark chocolate.

It is not only what they eat that sets French women apart from the rest of the world. If you want to fit in your trousers, you'd do well to steal another trick from them. It is simple: reduce the size of your portions. 'People tend to consume whatever is put in front of them,' says Professor Paul Rozin from the University of Pennsylvania, the co-author of the snappily entitled *The Ecology of Eating: Smaller Portion Sizes in France Than in the United States Help Explain the French Paradox.*

The French may no longer believe in god, but most of them still revere their cuisine. There is no such thing as a ready-made meal—unless it comes from their local *traiteur* whom they worship like their local priest and have known for years and trust to produce something fit for their dinner table.

11

Text Appeal

*'Woman knows not how to distinguish
her soul from her body.'*
Charles Baudelaire

A year after we moved to France, I joined a book
club. It was set up by another English woman
living in the area called Sue. She had put an advertisement in an English paper and my friend Carla (a former
literary editor, so obviously extremely intellectual)
suggested we go along. We sat in a room in the local
library, Sue, Carla and I with three other women. Two
Brits as well as one Hungarian who had lived in England
for almost twenty years.

Between us we decided which books to read and the

following month we met again to discuss one of our choices. The conversation was pretty straightforward.

Sue: 'What did you think of the book?'

Carla: 'Rubbish.' (I told you she was intellectual).

Me: 'I agree, crap.'

Daphne: 'I liked some of her other stuff but this one just didn't do it for me.'

After about ten minutes we would move on from talking about the book and the conversation would drift onto other things. Where to buy the best bread, for example, or a new bunch of expats that had moved into the region. Poor Sue would keep trying to bring us back to the book and we would make a half-hearted attempt to act interested but it didn't really work. We had a lovely time just gossiping.

All that changed the day the French arrived. Sue thought we were being too exclusively British so advertised the book club among the French community.

Suddenly we had to read books that were available in French as well. Our Wednesday afternoon meetings were taken over by French women who like nothing better than a seriously intellectual discussion. It was no longer enough to know who Albert Camus was, you now had to know his views on existentialism as well as his favourite colour. The soliloquies these women performed were enough to make Hamlet seem lost for words. I had no idea there were so many WORDS in the French language. Suddenly our very

English gathering had taken on a French slant, it had become intellectual.

W hereas in England it is embarrassing to be intellectual, in France it is essential. And the extraordinary thing is French women see intellectual rigour almost as important as their beauty regime.

It is not enough to look good to be seductive; you have to be cultured as well. At school if you take an academic baccalaureate, philosophy is a compulsory part of it. This teaches French school children to think in a way British ones don't. It gives them an intellectual advantage. Voltaire said of his mistress the Marquise du Châtelet: 'she was all passion, all mind'. All the French women I spoke to for this book said that a woman is sexy only if she is intelligent. 'For a French woman, humour, esprit and knowledge are much sexier than a short skirt and a pout,' says Florence Pernel. 'Men are attracted by a certain intellectual level.'

French women love going to anything remotely arty. They talk about the latest exhibition in much the same way English women would discuss the latest Robbie Williams single. On a recent trip to Paris, I went for a Sunday mid-morning walk. It was a glorious spring day, the streets were newly washed and Saint-Germain was sparkling. I came across a long queue on the rue de Grenelle. There must have been over a hundred people there, mainly women, from all age groups. Some with children, others alone or with friends, husbands or lovers. I thought maybe this was one of those famous designer discount sales which is one of the ways Parisians stay so scarily chic on a minimum budget.

I walked to the front of the queue. It turned out to be the entrance to the Musée Maillol: a charming museum that houses paintings and sculptures by a minor French artist, Aristide Maillol, whose main subject was female nudes. I asked an attractive woman in the queue if she often spent her Sundays queuing up for cultural events with her husband. She told me she went to something every weekend and that she would often queue for over two hours. 'For French women culture is almost as important as fashion,' she said. 'We see it as an essential part of our lives.' Although the British are famous for queuing, I can't imagine a similar scene in London, even for artistic nudes.

'France is more cultured,' says Michael Worton, Professor of French Literature at University College, London. 'They feel culture is much more important than we do.' The odd thing is I have found that since I moved to France I have grown more interested in museums. The Tate in London was not a place I was ever seen when I lived in London. Now I go every time I go back. It's become as necessary as a curry. Intellectuals in Britain have no real standing. There is a famous anecdote which illustrates this point. When Indira Gandhi was planning a visit to Britain in the 1980s, she wrote to Thatcher asking her to arrange a dinner with the top ten intellectuals in the country. Thatcher wrote back saying that in Britain there are no intellectuals. 'In contrast we live in a place where intellectuals still have a privileged place,' says the historian and psychoanalyst Elisabeth Roudinesco. 'The intellectuals in France can bring down a government. It has always been like this in France. Zola and Hugo for example were always at the forefront of politics.'

The *Académie Française* is further proof of the importance of intellectuals in France. This revered institution, founded in 1635, is the official guardian of the French language. Past members include Victor Hugo and Voltaire. The writers and intellectuals of the academy are responsible, among other things, for making sure not too much English sneaks into the French language. The members of the academy (forty in total) are known as *les immortels* (the immortals). They meet every week to debate the French language and add the fruits of the debate to the French dictionary. It is extremely hard to get in; you have to be a recognised writer, philosopher and generally seriously hot intellectual to stand any chance.

There have only ever been five female members of the

elite academy. Marguerite Yourcenar, the writer, was the first female member to be admitted. She was reading Racine and Aristophanes by the age of eight, she learnt Latin at ten and Greek at twelve. Just to give you some idea of the intellectual level we're talking here. The latest female member was admitted in June 2005. She is an Algerian author called Assia Djebar who writes about the lives of Muslim women.

Although I scoffed at the French cultural obsession at first, I now love the way they think and the fact that everyone here has an intellectual air about them.

I share my dog (a stray called Wolfie) with a neighbour, Madame Fonteneau. She is from an old wine-making family and is one of those formidable women you can imagine hiding English pilots during the war. She drives to the village in a bashed-up little van, normally wearing her apron and slippers. It is a look I am saving for my retirement years. Wolfie lives with us when it suits him and then wanders over to see Madame Fonteneau, who also feeds him and adores him. I saw her the other day and she asked if '*le chien loup*' as she calls him was with me. I said he was. She laughed and said: 'He is the personification of liberty.' I thought it was a wonderful and succinct description of him and wondered how many farmers' wives in England would describe a dog in terms one would normally reserve for a Marquis de Sade- type character.

The fact that culture is not just reserved for the elite is evident in the French TV schedule. A couple of years ago while British viewers watched Ulrika Johnson and her friends on Gladiators, French viewers watched Bernard Pivot—their version of Melvyn Bragg, including the riot of hair—and his panel of writers enjoy a battle of wits in a programme called *Bouillon de culture*. This programme was on French prime-time television, on a Friday night, and went on for *two* hours. And all they did was talk. Similarly, there is a mainstream channel here called Arte dedicated to culture, as well as a radio station called France Culture. Call anything culture or art in England and everyone will immediately hate it, and wonder why their money is being misspent on elitism.

I was on the train a few weeks ago; squashed into the corridor as there was some industrial action and only half the trains were running. With me were about fifteen people of all ages and all kinds of social backgrounds. There was a smart Parisian lady, a professional-looking gentleman type, a student, a middle-aged woman who I guessed was from the south by her looks and accent, a young woman, also from the south, travelling with her dog. Once we got moving, they all brought out their books. There was not one trashy novel among them (apart from mine of course). 'Chick-lit just doesn't happen in France,' says my friend Sebastian. 'The closest you get is something like *The Sexual Life of Catherine M*, sex glossed with an intellectual veneer.'

S ex as a subject is not taken lightly. Even *Emmanuelle*, which can really be described as porn, is filled with philosophy. 'It used to really annoy me when I was a teenager,' says Sebastian. 'I was keen to get back to the sex bits.' *Emmanuelle* is about a woman who goes to Thailand and has sex, a lot. The book, written by Emmanuelle Arsan (a pseudonym) was made into a film starring Sylvia Krystel and is probably still read by excited schoolboys all over the world.

When the film came out in 1974, it had a year-long run in Paris. Rather like the writer Colette, Emmanuelle is a woman who does what she wants, when she wants, with whomever she wants. A very French attitude.

And even Emmanuelle can't separate body and soul: 'When I have an orgasm, it's my spirit having an orgasm in my body; it's not my body returning to some earlier, bestial state! You want the spirit to take pleasure only in itself. Why? Life is wonderful throughout, in the flesh as well as the spirit.' The French certainly still take it seriously.

Watching the news after the Tsunami, I heard a French commentator saying that the fantasy of Emmanuelle in Thailand had been forever damaged by the tragedy.

Every aspect of sex is celebrated as a precious state of being. Take *The Piano Teacher* which came out a few years ago. OK, so it was based on a book written by an Austrian author, but this is not a film that would ever have been made in England or America for general release. It is about a frustrated and screwed-up piano teacher played by Isabelle Huppert. This is a woman who is so crazy she goes to peep shows and then mutilates her sex with a razor blade in her bathroom, as a sort of punishment.

She meets a gorgeous young student who falls madly in love with her. Instead of doing what any other sensible forty-year-old woman would do and having wild sex with him at every given opportunity, she demands from him that he beat her and go for sado-masochistic sex and weird mind games. Eventually she screws him up so much that he takes his revenge. I won't spoil the ending for you.

The French are big on watching sado-masochism. There are any number of classic films on the theme, of which *Belle de Jour* with Catherine Deneuve is probably the most famous. It starts with her being tied up to a tree, stripped to her underwear (matching of course) and whipped. I mean, how French is that? My babysitter Andrea and I watched it and afterwards she asked me if the DVD box came with a set of instructions.

All You Need to Be Impossibly French

Where Hollywood or English films thrive on plots and have to have one (much like Victorian paintings have a story), French films often don't really have a point. Not much happens, there's a lot of pontificating, some naked girls and strange music. Take *Breathless* in which Jean-Paul Belmondo plays a charming gangster in love with an American. They talk a lot, but don't really say anything. Conversation and events seem somehow random. Another classic is François Truffaut's *Jules et Jim*, which explores the famous French *ménage à trois*. It's a lovely film in lots of ways, atmospheric and dreamy, but try to explain the story and you're left wondering if there is one.

Jeanne Moreau, who stars in *Jules et Jim* is beautiful, even with a moustache. The film exposes another truth about French women; though they don't want to be men, they do like to dress up as them. Colette did it, George Sand did it. (But if you have a real moustache you're in trouble. Jeanette, my Montpellier friend who is married to a Frenchman but comes from Yorkshire originally, says she had a moustache when she first moved here. 'My husband's family all used to call me *el gringo*,' she tells me. 'After a while I asked them what they do about moustaches and they told me they waxed them, so that's what I do now.')

Even when they try to do real porn, they have to intellectualise it. I was reading a copy of the French *Glamour* magazine recently. There was an article entitled 'My best ever night of sex'. Sitting in a packed train I was a little embarrassed to be reading such smut, but obviously carried on anyway. One of the stories was written by a woman in her early twenties who had gone on a beach holiday with her boyfriend and best friend. The boyfriend went to bed early one night, leaving said girl and friend to go out alone. They run across some hunk and end up in a threesome on the beach—like you do. It made for a great read. Imagine my surprise though when at the end of her salacious description there was some psychiatrist analysing her best-ever night. 'This woman is clearly in love with her girlfriend,' writes the shrink. 'She never once mentions the stranger's penis.'

In France it doesn't seem possible to talk, write or have sex just for the sake of it. There always has to be an intellectual element to it. Maybe this is because French women argue seduction has almost as much to do with the mind as it does their looks; as much to do with her ability to quote Baudelaire as with her bra. She sees intelligence and knowledge as another accessory to complete her look and image.

There is an expression in France; *avoir du chien*. It means to be sexy, attractive and brainy. To seduce a man you need to be able to make him laugh, entertain him and keep him interested. And it's not enough just to wear garters and have nice hair. You need to be able to go on to him about books as well. As Edith Wharton, the American author who lived in Paris and is buried at the American cemetery in Versailles says: 'The French are persuaded that the enjoyment of beauty and the exercise of critical intelligence are two of the best things worth living for.'

I asked all the women I spoke to for this book to name the French woman who has most inspired them as a role model. They almost all nominated writers or intellectuals.

Their lists starts with Simone de Beauvoir, the intellectual icon, in the fifth place. De Beauvoir was born into a respected bourgeois family in 1908. When she was twenty one, she moved to Paris to study philosophy at the Sorbonne. Subsequently she became one of the first women to be accepted to the *Ecole Normale Supérieure*, roughly the French equivalent of Oxford or Cambridge. She met the philosopher Jean-Paul Sartre in 1928 and began a relationship with him that was to last until his death, although Sartre would be constantly unfaithful to her. A magazine article recently compared Angelina Jolie and Brad Pitt with Sartre and de Beauvoir. Clearly there is nothing remotely in common, but the French do like to glamorise their '*intellos*' (as they call them) and turn them into sex symbols.

De Beauvoir is most famous for her ground-breaking

feminist work *The Second Sex* published in 1949. In it she argues, among other things, that one isn't born a woman, one becomes one and that women can only be free outside the confines of the family. Her treatment of woman as the 'other' sex and the subsequent loss of social and personal identity is at the core of the book.

'She may not be so relevant to women today,' says Sylvie, my Montpellier friend who was one of the women who nominated de Beauvoir. 'But for me she is the beginning of real female emancipation in France. I also love the image of her and Sartre and their intellectual love affair, sitting in cafés in Paris, smoking and having heated discussions.' Anne Hidalgo, the renowned feminist who is number two at the mayor's office in Paris says of her 'she taught me not to accept the status of the second sex'. In the latest issue of *Elle* (obviously as a French woman I read 'the bible' as they call it every week) there is a fashion feature called 'Le Look Simone de Beauvoir.' 'The author of *The Second Sex* may have left us twenty years ago,' reads the stand-first. 'But her silhouette and her turban is always present.' There are pictures of her mixed and those of a model looking intellectual and elegant.

Simone de Beauvoir died in 1986 and was buried in the Cimetière de Montparnasse, in the same grave as Sartre. Feminists continue to complain that her name is under his. For those of you imagining they would be reunited in heaven, the atheist de Beauvoir will set you straight. 'My death will not bring us together again,' she wrote in *Adieux–A Farewell to Sartre*. 'This is how things are. It is in itself splendid that we are able to live our lives in harmony for so long.'

The fourth role model the French women mentioned was Louise de Vilmorin, one of the *grandes dames* of French literature and a socialite who was born into an aristocratic family in 1902. To learn more about her I went to visit Anne Marle, a cousin of François de Vilmorin, one of Louise's descendants, at the Sorbonne in Paris.

Anne, an elegant, small woman in her fifties meets me at the entrance gate. Like all great seats of learning there is something magical about the Sorbonne. We walk through the great court, towards her office on the second floor of the main building where she works as an historian. There is a great contrast between the elegant entrance and the shabby interior. The entrance hall is magnificent with arches leading off to various lecture halls like the Salle Richelieu. The floor is wooden and beautifully polished. In contrast, the little lift we take up to the second floor looks like one of those service lifts you get in big industrial buildings.

We sit down in her office and Anne tells me the story of Louise de Vilmorin. She was born in the family château just outside Paris. In 1923 she was briefly engaged to Antoine de Saint-Exupéry, author of *The Little Prince*. But she broke his heart when she called off the engagement. Her first husband was the American property heir Henry

Leigh-Hunt, whom she would later describe as '*cet odieux Monsieur Leigh-Hunt*'. They married in 1925 and had three daughters. She left him after a stint in his home city of Las Vegas (probably not the ideal place for a sensitive and literary French aristocrat). She also had a fling with Orson Welles and was married twice again, once to a Hungarian count and finally to the French culture minister André Malraux.

But it is her *ménage à trois* with Duff Cooper, the British Ambassador to Paris and his wife Diana that she is most famous for. Duff Cooper, who translated her most celebrated novel *Madame De* into English, was her lover for several years. It is said his beautiful wife Diana was as mad about de Vilmorin as he was. Her biographer, Jean Botherel, says: 'The three were bound together in a strange harmony, mysterious and incomprehensible to all their friends... They loved each other.... Their correspondence leaves absolutely no doubt as to the extraordinary equilibrium in the relations between them. When Duff was absent, Diana was the only person Louise wanted to be with. She loved her with a real tenderness and wrote her burning poems.'

'She was a great seductress,' says Anne. 'People fell in love with her. She had a great power over men, which she cultivated from an early age in the relationship with her four brothers. The relationship is slightly ambiguous, they were all crazy about each other.'

Though practically unknown anywhere else, in France she is one of the most popular female icons. 'She just had it all,' says my friend Nathalie. 'She was beautiful, elegant, cultivated and part of the intellectual jet-set. A sort of literary 'It' girl.' Charlotte, my publishing friend agrees. 'She was the classic Parisian,' she says. 'Witty and pretty, very intelligent and extremely frivolous at the same time.'

Wonderful as she was, she was unable to mesmerise everyone. In a letter to Nancy Mitford, Evelyn Waugh describes her as 'a Hungarian countess who pretended to be a French poet. An egocentric maniac with the eyes of a witch. She is the spirit of France. How I hate the French.' Mitford agrees. 'Oh how glad I am you felt this about Loulou (Louise's nickname)—I can't sit in a room with her, she makes me so nervous. And vicious. She is much more like a middle European than a French woman.' Anne disagrees. 'She is so very French,' she says. 'You can feel her elegance in her writing. The strange thing is she was never really sophisticated, she had more of an instinctive intelligence and confidence. And although I would describe her as gifted, I wouldn't say she was intellectual.'

I agree with that. I have read her most famous book *Madame De* and found it extremely forgettable. The version I read was translated by her lover Duff Cooper, so you would think if there was any passion in the original he would have picked up on it. It was stylised, shallow, and I felt hardly any sympathy for the heroine. It seems culture for French women is a little like their underwear; nicely put together but easy to take on and off.

George Sand, the number three, was a more serious woman. Unlike Louise she wasn't blessed with natural beauty, but was still a great seducer and famous for her passionate affairs with contemporary stars like the composer Chopin, the French Romantic poet Alfred de Musset and the dramatist Prosper Mérimée, author of the novella *Carmen* that inspired the opera by Bizet.

George Sand was born Amantine Aurore Lucille Dupin in Paris on 1 July 1804. She was the daughter of an aristocratic father and a mother from humble origins. She married young and left her unfaithful husband to pursue a career as a journalist in Paris. She took her two children with her and supported the family through writing. She got a job on *Le Figaro* via an introduction from one of her lovers and would show up to work dressed as a man. Some say it was because she wanted to be taken seriously, others because she had no money to dress herself properly. She also adopted the pseudonym George Sand so that her work would not be immediately looked at as belonging to a woman.

'My profession is to be free,' she said, and with the publication of her novel *Indiana* in 1832 she finally earned enough money to be independent. Although she wrote seventy novels, twenty four plays and over forty thousand letters, she is really more remembered for her insistence that women should be as free as men to pursue their lives and loves. 'I ask the support of no one,' she said. 'Neither to kill someone for me, gather a bouquet, correct a proof, nor to go with to the theatre. I go there on my own, as a man, by choice; and when I want flowers, I go on foot, by myself, to the Alps.'

She was also famous for being part of an intellectual set which included the painter Eugène Delacroix, Balzac and Liszt, as well as the great love of her life, Frédéric Chopin. She would entertain them all in her country house, where she stayed up most of the night writing, rising at midday to spend the afternoons with her friends before going back to her desk. Her affair with Chopin ended when she suspected that he had fallen in love with her daughter Solange.

My friend Anne at the Sorbonne says that if Sand had stayed with her husband she would never have become such an important figure. 'If he had made her happy, there would have been no George Sand,' she said. To George Sand there was nothing as important as love. 'There is only one happiness in life,' she says. 'To love and be loved.'

George Sand died in 1876. 'The world will know and understand me someday,' Sand once wrote. 'But if that day does not arrive, it does not greatly matter. I shall have opened the way for other women.'

Anne says her novels make dreary reading nowadays but her image is what is important and inspiring. 'Some of her works are charming, of course,' she says. 'But they are old-fashioned. What we take from her is the image of a free woman who loves life and is determined to fight for her liberty in every sense of the word.'

The runner-up is Françoise Sagan, who became famous at the age of eighteen with the publication of the brilliant novel on teenage angst *Bonjour Tristesse*. I first read it in my early twenties on the beach in Italy. I immediately identified with the heroine Cécile, who has a good-looking, philandering father. My father was the same. It is a short book (always a good start) and one that should be read in one sitting if possible. It engulfs you and I defy anyone not to be touched by it. The five million people worldwide who have bought it must be on to something.

Sagan was born Françoise Quoirez in 1935 in the Lot, south-west France, to a prosperous, bourgeois family. She was educated in convent schools and the Sorbonne. She wrote *Bonjour Tristesse* in the bistros around the Sorbonne during her seven-week summer break. When she told her father it was going to be published, he forbade her from using the family name, so she adopted a name from a character in Proust.

When I visit Anne at the Sorbonne, I have lunch in one of the bistros in the little square outside the university. There are students everywhere, sitting on the pavements, on the fountain in the middle of the little square, all chatting, reading and eating their lunch. I imagine the young Sagan sitting there writing her most famous novel.

She wrote another thirty novels but none achieved the success of the first.

Her work was criticised by some as being too elitist. She wrote mainly against a backdrop of casinos, fast cars, racehorses and rich older men. And although she was very much part of the famous French existentialist intellectual scene of Saint-Germain, some critics questioned her right to belong to it. She responded by saying that it was the only world she knew. 'It would be bad form for me to describe people I don't know and I don't understand,' she said. 'Think about it. Whisky, Ferraris and gambling; aren't they rather more amusing than knitting, housekeeping and one's savings?'

Sagan's life was never trouble free. She was thrown out of the Sorbonne for failing her exams, she took drugs and she was convicted of defrauding the French tax authorities a couple of years before she died. Her property had been seized, her racehorses sold and her sports cars gone. She died a pauper in 2004. One of the women who nominated her was Sabbia Rosa who told me why she loves *Bonjour Tristesse*. 'When it came out in 1954, I had just lost my father, so I related to the heroine and her fear,' she says. 'It is the book that has touched me most in my life, filled with tenderness, sadness and melancholy.'

One of the most beautiful squares in Paris is the Place Colette. It is in the exclusive first arrondissement, close to the Louvre and the Palais Royal. The square is lined with classically French buildings. On a plaque is written 'Place Colette Sidonie-Gabrielle Colette 1873-1954 Romancière Française.' It is a fitting tribute to the woman who was mentioned most as the quintessential French woman, Colette.

Just the name conjures up images of debauchery and naughtiness. She is undoubtedly one of the most formidable of French women, one outstandingly talented and raucous character.

She was born in Burgundy in 1873. Her father was a retired army officer and her mother was a radical character who shocked the village by refusing to wear mourning clothes when her husband died. At the age of twenty Colette married the music critic Henri Gauthier-Villars (Willy) and set up home in Paris. He was a writer of trashy novels and fifteen years older than her. He was interested in the stories of her school life and encouraged her to write them down. Thus the Claudine novels were born, which he published under his own name and which made him rich and famous. Colette didn't much care for writing and so Willy would lock her in a room until she had written enough pages.

When she left him, Colette tried to make a living from her books but found she couldn't. She became a music hall dancer, while writing on various topics for newspapers. In 1910 she wrote *Renée* which was an immediate success. In 1920 she wrote what is probably her most famous novel, *Chéri*, the story of an ageing courtesan and her young lover. She is best known in England and America for *Gigi* which was dramatized for Broadway and also made into a film. The play made Audrey Hepburn (who was personally chosen by Colette) a star.

'I love Colette, all her work; when I write she is the only one I can read,' says the French novelist Anny Duperey. 'She is an example of a woman who uses her sensuality to write. She has an extraordinary intelligence, an attention to detail and scalpel-like precision.'

Michael Worton describes Colette as one of the most important figures in French literature. 'The extraordinary thing about France is that although their education encourages conformity, you then have people like Colette who inspire confidence and individuality,' he says. 'Here is a woman who starts off locked in a room by Willy, then gets one over on all her men, marries her son-in-law, dances half-naked on tables as a grand old dame and writes terribly well about the transgressive love between an older woman and a younger man. She was so incredibly herself.'

Of all the women on the list, Colette is my favourite. She was a very daring character whose life was dominated by the sensual. If anyone has succeeded in leaving French women with an image of a free, libertine, successful and sexy role model, it is Colette. And quite apart from anything else, her books are a very good read. They are simply written but she can convey a whole mood in a few words.

All these women have one thing in common though: they are glamorous. Even George Sand, who was, as Anne Marle puts it, 'quite ugly', was a great seductress and therefore automatically seen as attractive. They are also all free. They take lovers when they want to, get drunk or high if they feel like it and drive fast cars. They behave like men. Maybe it's thanks to George Sand they are able to.

I try to imagine a similar list of British female icons. First I don't think British women would choose literary role models. I think we would have Marianne Faithful, maybe Margaret Thatcher or worse. One English girl I met at a wedding here said Kate Bush was her heroine. I wanted to ask her why but just didn't have the energy.

If you look at literary role models such as Virginia Woolf, Emily Brontë, Jane Austen or George Eliot, none of them had the exciting and free lives the French did. And not one of them is a famous seductress. Most of them probably died virgins. At any rate two of them died unmarried.

There are some twentieth century British examples to compare with Sagan and Colette. Iris Murdoch's first published work in 1953 was called *Sartre, Romantic Rationalist,* so she was at least part of the gang. And she did apparently have lots of affairs. But she was always a hippy-like type with greasy hair and hardly a sexual icon. In a recent posthumous book her lover Elias Cannetti wrote that sex with her wasn't very good and she wore large grey panties. Doris Lessing is another great writer, but not sexy. The American poet Sylvia Plath was undeniably glamorous and her association with the English poet Ted Hughes was passionate and dramatic. But as she killed herself, she can hardly be a role model for women today.

W̲e don't have the same heritage of strong, sexy and intellectual women. I also don't think our cultural heritage is as important for most of us as it is for the French. Maybe it's an educational factor, the education here is very academic, so most French women know a lot more about their literary past than their British equivalents. 'French women outclass their British and American equivalents by a huge margin in terms of education and conversation,' says a French male friend of mine who has lived in all three countries. 'I always saw them as superior in that sense, although the downside is they are also a lot more difficult.'

I remember a French woman I once met at a party. She was a teacher and taught French literature. I asked her who her favourite female French writer was. She told me it was Colette. I asked her why. 'Because she had everything a French woman wants,' she told me. 'She had lots of husbands, lots of lovers and lots of confidence. Added to which she was incredibly intelligent and attractive.' It seems that as with everything in France, culture is linked with the sensual. Colette once received a letter from a critic. 'Can't you possibly write a book that isn't about love or adultery or separation, or some other semi-incestuous affair? Isn't there anything else in life?'

Not in France there isn't. Apart from food that is.

12

Dangerous Liaisons

*'When she raises her eyelids, it's as if she
were taking off all her clothes.'*
Colette

It is Nadine, my English friend who lives in Paris, who first tells me about the shop. 'I have a huge thing to tell you about French women,' she emails me one day. 'The big thing *entre femmes chics* is Sonia Rykel's sex shop in the rue de Grenelle where the most bourgeois French women spend $365 on... well you'll have to see for yourself.'

I have just had a meeting with a marvellous lady at the Sorbonne and have an hour before my next one. I decide it's an ideal opportunity to see what Nadine is on about. I am expecting a proper sex shop, vibrators in the window, videos with nasty looking Germans shouting obscenities, the normal kind of thing. I am almost nervous to give the taxi driver the address in case he thinks I'm a pervert.

Imagine my surprise then when he tells me we've arrived and I see an underwear shop. I go inside and there are lots of lovely little things for women like a pink silk bag to put one's mobile phone in and an exquisite jewellery case in pink satin and black velvet. But not a dildo in sight. There is an immaculate sales assistant standing at the bottom of some stairs. I ask her if I can go upstairs. 'Yes,' she says smilingly. 'I'll come with you.' Now you're talking. I go upstairs expecting to find a haven of sex toys and blow-up dolls. Not a bit of it. It's full of underwear. For the bargain price of $550 I can kit myself out in silk. I try on a couple of camisoles, just to make sure the sex toys aren't hidden in the changing room and then go back downstairs. It's as I am leaving that I see a big sign hanging over the stairs that lead to the basement. '*Interdit aux mineurs*' it reads.

'Oh,' I say, trying to sound totally surprised. 'Is there a downstairs?'

'Yes,' says Miss Immaculate. '*Ca c'est les sex toys.*'

'Oh,' I say again, feigning nonchalance. 'I might take a look.'

'Help yourself, my colleague is downstairs.' Wearing rubber I assume.

I go down into the basement which is much darker than the rest of the shop and decorated in black. It is rather like a bat cave. There is a couple down there choosing something, but good manners prevent me from prying and I develop a sudden interest in cashmere dressing gowns I could never afford. Finally they leave, having decided that the man will come back later and buy whatever it is as a surprise for the woman.

Solenn is my guide to the dark and mysterious world of Sonia Rykel sex toys. She is about two metres tall, very pretty, dressed entirely in black (cotton not rubber) and thinner than anyone I have ever met. She wears rather sober glasses and looks more like a schoolteacher than a sex-toy expert as she guides me through the various options.

'Over here we have the external stimulation division,' she sweeps an arm across some very odd-looking things which I assume vibrate. 'And over here the internal stimulation.' Each item is exquisitely displayed on a glass tray; it's more like choosing a piece of priceless porcelain than a vibrator.

Solenn goes on to explain that the most popular models of internal stimulation are the pink one, affectionately named stubby, and the rabbit. 'The pink is the optimum shape and size for reaching the g-spot,' she tells me. 'It vibrates and also stimulates the outside.' She turns it on. 'As you can hear, it's very quiet.'

Stubby retails at the bargain price of $165. The rabbit is

cheaper (only $125) but is much noisier and somehow less exquisite. Trust the French to make the question of elegance an issue when buying sex toys. The rabbit is see-through red rubber with coloured beads inside which are apparently very stimulating. It has a fork-shaped contraption which caresses the clitoris. 'Women I have spoken to who have used it say there's nothing better,' says Solenn.

I ask Solenn which she thinks is the best one. 'I've no idea,' she says. 'I haven't tried them.' (I'm not sure I believe her. I mean, stuck in that basement all day, you'd just have to, wouldn't you?) 'But,' she continues in her businesslike manner, rather like she is describing the pros and cons of a washing machine, 'the pink is waterproof. You can't actually take it in the bath but it can be used in the shower which is good when it comes to cleaning. And it is somehow less mechanical looking, a little more romantic. Also I do believe that on maximum speed the rabbit can be a little too much.'

We move onto the fur wraps sold in the basement. They are gorgeous, and start at $900. I am briefly tempted but go upstairs to talk some more to Miss Immaculate. 'The idea behind the shop was to create a place where women could come just for their pleasure,' she says. 'A place that wasn't seedy but was luxurious and elegant. A place where sex toys are no longer seen as taboo but as part of the pleasure that a woman can have, like the underwear we sell or the little luxury items.'

Sex and seduction, is part of everyday life in France. 'In France, women have always wanted to seduce men,' Charlotte Rampling, who lives in France, said in a recent interview with the *Sunday Times*. 'But not really in England. In France seduction is part of the culture, like wine and cheese.'

The culture element is crucial. Writers like Colette, George Sand and Louise de Vilmorin inspire women of today in their behaviour and belief that they can have it all. French women certainly have better examples than we Brits have from literature. While George Sand was trying to get laid, Emily Brontë was fictionalising her sexual hero in *Wuthering Heights*. While Emma Bovary was in the back of a carriage with the young Léon, Elisabeth Bennet was trying to bag a suitable husband.

As my friend Aurélie says: 'Our culture of *l'amour libertin* is a heritage we cannot avoid. We have grown up with books like *Dangerous Liaisons* and characters like the Marquis of Sade and Colette. They are part of our education.'

French women are sexy, there is no denying it. They have a certain way of talking to men, of holding their heads, smiling and charming them. There is a great word in French; *coquine*. It is often used with little girls when they are being very sweet but a little naughty. *Elle fait la coquine*, they say. I think grown women do it too, almost all the time.

'French women are programmed to seduce,' says Alexandre, a male French friend of mine who lives in the Dordogne. This statement prompted me to ask an English friend of mine what she thought English women were programmed to do. 'Cuddle their dogs,' was her response. For the French woman, seduction permeates everyday life. This is the reason she always needs to look good.

So are they better in bed than English women? Is it purely by accident that the phrase *femme fatale* is a French one? Henry VIII had a French mistress and was extremely impressed with her. In his diary he wrote about the delightful times he spent with Marie. 'We hid sweetmeats in our private parts, to be extracted, as was our rule, only by the tongue, never by the fingers... I entered her and we turned the sandglass and counted how many times we could come to culmination, both together and separately. Then I decked her naked body with my wife's jewels and mounting her among the precious gems felt the most adulterous of all. Expertly she swam under me bringing me to *la petite morte* several times in succession. This is yet another admirable French talent, as no *femme fatale* worth of her name is satisfied with only one orgasm—no there must be a series for both, the more the better. Such exercises and flattery were only the beginning of her artful French repertoire. There were many things that decency does not permit me to record, even in my own private book.'

My friend James's first ever girlfriend was French and a

few years older than him. He met her when he was sixteen and on holiday with his parents in Provence. He had been back at school for three weeks when the headmaster summoned him to his office. 'There is a young lady here to see you,' he said. 'And she appears to be French.' Since then James has never looked back.

He finds French women much sexier. 'In my experience French women are better in bed than English women. English women tend to know what they need to pleasure themselves and pay little attention to the man's needs,' he says, 'whereas French women are fully engrossed in giving and receiving pleasure. French women are also a lot more adventurous when it comes to positions and when to have sex. The English, I think, are a lot more conservative, which is quite strange when one looks at how much easier English women are to get into the sack than their French counterparts.'

Another male friend of mine who wishes to remain nameless but has a French mistress says that French women seem to worship the penis in a way English women don't. 'They just adore it. There is no sense of smuttiness attached to their relationship with a penis. It's a natural thing,' he says. 'And this makes them more adventurous lovers. They seem more at ease with it and eager to get their hands on it.'

Charles, a wine-making friend of mine who lived with a French woman for ten years, says he finds their open attitude to sex a little disconcerting. 'I am shocked by the graphic terms they use to describe men, the way they discuss everything from penis size to how they perform in bed with each other, totally with no holds barred. Maybe it's an indication that they're not as oppressed as the Brits but it can sound a little vulgar.'

For French women, sex and seduction are part of a repertoire that ensures her success and social standing. They seduce everyone. Not literally, but it is important to them that men adore them. A French woman may only be seducing the bus driver on the way to work, or the man in the café who brings her morning *café au lait*, but the ability to do so is paramount and a vital part of her self esteem.

For French men it is an essential part of daily life too. 'This sexy rapport is one of the reasons I love it here and could never move back,' says my friend Jeanette. 'Men here are not afraid to look at you, to chat you up and it is generally accepted that women use their charms to get what they want. When I go back to England, I feel very lonely; no one looks at me any more, it's just like I'm alone in a world of molecules knocking together, there is nothing chemical going on, no exchanges or interaction.'

Jeanette is adamant she would have more chance of securing a bank loan if her legs were waxed than if they weren't. 'People here like dealing with people that look good,' she says. 'There is no such word as no in the French language, it's just a question of degrees of no.'

French women may be programmed to seduce, but for some of them it is more serious. Seduction is essential. Agnès Cromback tells me about a friend of hers who has a constant need to seduce. 'One of my friends really has a need to stray,' she says. 'This need is stronger than her. She has a great job, a husband and children, but this thing is completely apart. In her head she doesn't think she's doing anything wrong.'

I ask Agnès if she condemns her friend's behaviour.

'Intellectually it shocks me that she is being unfaithful to her husband but on the other hand seducing young men is her way of functioning. What worries me is how she will stop, because she has to stop one day. She can't go on forever seducing more and more, she will end up a ridiculous figure.'

Their culture has given French women independence and a taste for freedom. If you cut a French woman in half, you will see the words *liberté, egalité, fraternité* written throughout like a stick of rock. And of these the most important is *liberté*. As Michael Worton says: 'The whole notion of freedom is deeply inscribed in the French psyche. Marrying and then misbehaving is seen as being free.'

The French differ hugely from the Brits and Americans when it comes to fidelity. The French view adultery as a fairly normal pastime. 'It's one of the two favourite sports in France, the other being eating,' says Henri my French male friend. The writer Alexandre Dumas said: 'The chain of wedlock is so heavy it takes two to carry it, sometimes three.'

I meet Charlotte, a very pretty Parisian friend of mine who works in publishing, to discuss illicit romance and other topics. What better place to discuss infidelity than the Café de Flore on the Boulevard Saint-Germain? This is the legendary café where the womaniser Sartre and his long-suffering partner Simone de Beauvoir used to meet. Charlotte and I are discussing '*les petites aventures*' as the French call them.

'They're not so very serious,' she says. 'I don't think people really mind them.'

'Mind them?' I am incredulous. 'My husband told me he would sleep with the babysitter if I ever have an affair.' This is something I cannot risk. Good babysitters are hard to find.

Now it is Charlotte's turn to look incredulous. 'But you don't have to tell him,' she says, taking another sip of her green tea.

It is not until later that day when I get a text message from B that I have to ask myself the question of whether I have now become so French that I will stray. 'If you are in Paris tonight I am in a suite at the Meurice,' it reads. I am indeed in Paris and booked to stay the night, in a rather charming if down-market hotel called the Hôtel Pas de Calais. A suite at the five-star Meurice with the enigmatic B sounds far more exciting than listening to the German guests next door planning their next day's sightseeing. And would my husband ever find out?

Charlotte is not the only French woman who thinks affairs are justifiable, if carried out with discretion. I meet one lady who shall remain nameless who tells me that she had been having affairs with guys at work for the last three years. I ask if her husband knows or if she felt guilty.

'Of course he doesn't know,' she tells me. 'Why would he want to? I'm much happier this way so he is too.'

I'm not sure her husband would agree with her. Although French men see little wrong in having a mistress. A good male friend of ours even discussed whether one should address one's mistress with the formal *vous* or the informal *tu*. 'I find *vous* much sexier,' he said. And this was in front of his wife. According to him around eighty per cent of his male friends are unfaithful. And there can't just be a stock of single women out there, so it figures a lot of married women are enjoying a bit of side-salad too.

As B points out to me, adultery among politicians is always forgiven. His female compatriots agree with him. 'We think it's a good thing for the nation if the President has sex with a little intern,' says the actress Florence Pernel. 'Because if a man doesn't have sex he is terrible. Chirac has had hundreds of affairs.' Hermine is astounded that President Clinton felt the need to tell the nation about it. 'It's his sex life,' she says. 'He only owes an explanation to his wife, not to the whole of America. It's completely bizarre.' The actress Anny Duperey agrees. 'It's like something from Mars,' she says. 'The man had a blow-job, so what? In France we would fall over in the street if our politicians started apologising for their sex lives.'

Mitterrand famously led a double life for years, even fathering a child with another woman. At his funeral it was the image of his widow and mistress together in mourning that made it to the front pages of all the papers. But what shocked the French most was not the fact that he had been unfaithful but the fact that he had lied about his daughter for so long. 'We would have welcomed the little girl, treasured her,' says the Sorbonne historian Anne Marle. 'We would have forgiven everything, but not the lie.'

People in France are worried that the Puritanism we have in Britain and America is coming their way. 'For us it would be the end of civilization,' says the historian and psychoanalyst Elisabeth Roudinesco. 'The fact that a politician in England doesn't have the right to a mistress is ridiculous. Humans are made of complicated things. You cannot make man pure, man is made of passion. If you try for purity you will have misery, just look at the US. The state should not get involved in people's private lives and people should not be judged according to their sex lives, as long as they are within the law.'

French literature and history is of course full of examples of faithless wives. Zola's doomed heroine Thérèse Raquin for example. Eleanor of Aquitaine cuckolded her husband Louis VII during the second crusade with one of her uncles. The king tried to cover up the scandal but once back in France he divorced her. So she went to England and was 'consoled' by Henri II.

The most famous of all unfaithful French women must be Flaubert's Madame Bovary, the innocent young doctor's wife who is betrayed by her own yearning for true love and unrealised dreams. Like many French women I spoke to who were having affairs, she seems able to distinguish the two lives pretty effectively. This is a conversation between her and her lover Léon.

'When they talked of Paris, she often ended by murmuring, 'How happy we could be there!'

'Aren't we happy?' the young man asked gently, stroking her hair.

'Yes, of course,' she said, 'I'm being silly. Kiss me!'

To her husband she was more charming than ever, making him pistachio-creams and playing him waltzes after dinner. He thought himself, in consequence, the luckiest of mortals.'

Of course it all ends badly for Emma, mainly due to her choice of men. But even if she didn't get to live life in the way it is described in the books she avidly reads, Madame Bovary has made it into one. She is in the French dictionary. There is a noun, *bovarysme*, which means a tendency to romanticise reality as a way of escaping the limitations of one's own existence.

The painful example of Emma Bovary's downfall does not stop French women straying. According to a survey carried out by *Institut français d'opinion publique* of 410 women aged between eighteen and thirty nine about fidelity of women while in holiday, only two per cent of them said they would not consider being unfaithful. Most of them (forty four per cent) said they would pick a man who was amusing above everything else and sixty seven per cent said their preferred place for illicit sex was the beach. The sea was the next favourite spot.

Anne Marle says French infidelity has a lot to do with their Catholic upbringing. 'It is forbidden so it is very exciting,' she says. 'The delicious taste of sin. Then of course you just say sorry, which is another form of seduction.' I ask Geneviève de Fontenay if she thinks the French are more prone to misbehaviour than the English.

'No,' she says. 'We have our *cinq à sept*, but you have your tea. *C'est la même chose je suppose*—the same, I guess?'

So how do French women justify their infidelity? I speak to one young lady who lives outside Lyon. She has been cheating on her husband for three months with a friend of theirs. 'I don't feel guilty at all,' she tells me. 'My husband just doesn't give me what I want any more, he doesn't notice me. He's always in front of his computer. My lover is tender and kind and passionate.'

A friend of mine from Paris is also having an affair. She justifies it by saying that her husband enjoys all the new underwear she buys to seduce her lover with. He may not like it so much if he knew he was the second man to enjoy it that day. But French women don't seem to care. For them anything is excusable if they're in love. No one will condemn them; in fact they are more likely to condemn unfulfilled love. Love and lust excuse any conduct.

For men having a mistress carries no stigma, rather it is an advantage as it shows you have money and status. But what do French women do if their husbands are unfaithful? I am told a story by a friend of mine who lives outside Toulouse. A wife in his village has just found out her husband has been unfaithful to her. He has been sleeping with the woman at the local post office. They live in a rural area and have been married for seven years. They have two children. The wronged wife goes to see a friend and asks if she can borrow his house. 'What for?' says the friend.

'I need somewhere we can be alone. I want to seduce my husband,' replies the wronged wife.

I may be wrong, but I would guess that the first reaction of most English and American women on discovering their husband's infidelity would not be to treat him to a sex session. But this is exactly what this French woman in the Midi-Pyrénées did. She seduced her philandering husband in the house of her friend. The outcome was that he came back to her, although only for a few months (the post office mistress proved too much of a temptation).

The husband in this story broke one of the cardinal rules of playing around: discretion. Going for someone in the same village is not good manners. It humiliates your wife, which is seen as extremely un-gentlemanly, in a way that sleeping with someone else simply isn't. Logical? Maybe not, but I can see their point.

Brigitte Bardot famously broke the cardinal rule of discretion when she had an affair with Serge Gainsbourg. They met in 1968 when she was married to the German millionaire Gunther Sachs. They fell madly in love and began an affair. During their affair they recorded the first and steamiest version of *Je t'aime moi non plus*. Sachs and Bardot convinced Gainsbourg not to release the single. He eventually re-recorded it with Jane Birkin.

Also along the discretion theme, if there is a split between lovers, the public must not know about it. In her novel *Madame De*, Louise de Vilmorin describes the following scene after the Ambassador has split up with the heroine.

'The Ambassador was henceforth so careful to do nothing in public to offend her vanity that nobody suspected there was any change in his feelings towards her.'

The Paris-based American author Edith Kunz says the whole system works rather well. 'Wives, husbands, mistresses and lovers function together on a relatively peaceful basis in France when the players adhere to the nonverbal code of manners,' she says. 'Statistics of spousal homicide and abuse register forty per cent lower in France than in the United States.'

As I wander back to Saint-Germain I walk past the Hotel Meurice. Somewhere up there in a suite is an attractive French man waiting to undress me. His presence in Paris has made my research so much more exciting and fun. Ever since I first met him on the train I have been thinking about what it would be like to kiss him. I have never had a foreign lover; could he be the one that changes this?

I stop outside the door of the hotel. All I have to do is go in and ask for him. Within minutes I'll be in his suite drinking champagne and showing off my new underwear. I have goose-pimples at the thought of it. Then another thought strikes me.

I realise that actually turning B into a lover in the physical sense is not what I want. What I enjoy about having him around is the idea of a lover. I like the idea of being attractive to him; it motivates me to look after myself. I like having a flirtation but I think if it were to go beyond that it could all go horribly wrong. As Coco Chanel said: 'Elegance is refusal.'

All You Need to Be Impossibly French

I have learned from French women and their attitude to love is that if you don't have a lover, you should always behave as if you do. Always be ready and presentable enough to be seen naked (or in matching underwear) by the man of your fantasies, even if he stays just that.

My Year in Training

This is a French joke.

Question: What do you call a pretty girl in London?

Answer: A tourist.

The French still believe we Brits and Americans have no idea how to look good. They see us as amusing but rather inept when it comes to putting on a dress.

They have a point. I have been impressed with the French women I met for this book. They are beautiful, intelligent and elegant. If it needed doing, I can confirm that French women have a lot of style.

So what is their secret? Sophie told me all those years ago that all you need to be French is two lipsticks and a lover. Not true. You need a lot more. You need an iron will to resist any (edible) temptation that comes your way. You need to be able to make a little time for yourself every day and spend some money on your beauty regime. You also need to find an excellent hairdresser and a good manicurist. You need to make your body, face and style a priority. And then you are ready to start reading Colette and Flaubert.

I am happy about the way in which I have changed since we moved here. I am thinner, healthier and perhaps more stylish. During a recent trip to Paris a courier stopped me on his bike outside the Louvre to ask me for directions. I have rarely been more flattered; to be mistaken for a French woman is one thing. To be mistaken for a Parisian is more than I could have hoped for.

I do look different now. I probably act a little differently too. But the thing that has surprised me is that I am not really doing this for anyone else. I have become used to being like this and I can't go back now. It makes me feel good. Even if no one is going to see my underwear, it always has to be matching or I feel clumsy and wrong.

There is, however, a downside to the French obsession with beauty.

Here is my version of the joke I began with.

Question: What do you call a girl who is having a good time in Paris?

Answer: A tourist.

I was meeting a French male friend of mine for dinner in Paris recently. I called him and asked him if I could bring someone with me.

'Yes, of course,' he said. 'As long as she's not French.'

When I asked him to explain why he told me he was sick of going out with French women. 'They are dreadful company,' he said. 'They don't eat, they don't drink and they don't laugh: they are too busy thinking about how they look to relax. It drives me insane.'

Is the truth that French women are thin and perfect looking, but don't have much fun? Maybe. They are working so hard to be perfect, they never seem to stop to enjoy the way they are. Being born a French woman has its advantages, but it also comes with a huge responsibility. You have a reputation to live up to.

I am going to take what is useful from their way of life (and there is a lot) but stay fundamentally English. If this means drinking a bit too much Chardonnay at times or not having perfect nails three hundred and sixty five days a year, so be it.

My husband says the key is to 'keep your sense of humour but still be able to fit into your trousers'. Sounds like a good plan to me.

And obviously I'll be wearing garters and matching underwear underneath.

Acknowledgements

A huge thank you to all the French women who helped me with this book. They were all extremely generous with their time, secrets and tips. I was touched at how welcoming they were and how willing they were to help me. A special thank you to the inspirational (and very thin) Inès de la Fressange, the first person I interviewed for this book. Thank you also to all the men who took time to talk to me about French women, a subject that is never dull. Thanks as always to Jacques Kuhnlé for his meticulous research and reading. Thank you to my publisher Martin Rynja for his support and diligence and to Mary Jones for her help with publicity. Many thanks as always to Jonathan Miller for brilliant sound bites and sexing up. Thank you also to Carla McKay, who reminded me why English women are such fun. Most of all thank you to Rupert, my husband and favourite editor, who put up with me obsessing about the book for months. He now knows more about face creams than any other Englishman. And of course, underwear. There have to be some perks.